Reiki

ENERGY MEDICINE

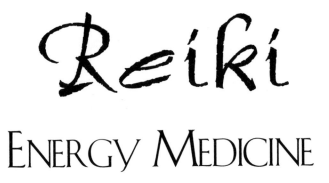

ENERGY MEDICINE

BRINGING HEALING TOUCH INTO HOME, HOSPITAL, AND HOSPICE

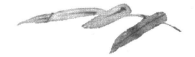

LIBBY BARNETT AND MAGGIE CHAMBERS

WITH SUSAN DAVIDSON

Healing Arts Press
Rochester, Vermont

Healing Arts Press
One Park Street
Rochester, Vermont 05767
www.InnerTraditions.com

Healing Arts Press is a division of Inner Traditions International

Note to reader: The stories in this book are based on the actual experiences of real people. Some are composite histories. All names have been changed to preserve privacy. This book is not intended to give advice for the treatment of particular illnesses. It is an examination of Reiki as an adjunctive therapy to conventional medical approaches. It is suggested that the reader seek the expertise of a trained healthcare professional to treat any serious ailment.

In all cases the publisher and authors have made every effort to contact and get permission from the people appearing in this book. If omissions or errors have occurred, we encourage you to contact Inner Traditions International.

LIBRARY OF CONGRESS CATALOGING-IN-PUBLICATION DATA

Barnett, Libby
      Reiki energy medicine : bringing healing touch into home, hospital, and hospice / Libby Barnett and Maggie Chambers, with Susan Davidson.
         p.   cm.
         Includes bibliographical references.
         ISBN 0-89281-633-3
         1. Reiki (Healing stystem)   I. Chambers, Maggie   II. Davidson, Susan.
III. Title.
RZ403.R45B37   1996
615.8'52—dc20

                                               96-3962
                                               CIP

Printed and bound in Canada

10 9 8 7

Typesetting and layout by Charlotte Tyler
This book was typeset in Schneidler with Ruling Script Two as a display typeface
Photographs and illustrations by Maggie Chambers, except page 62, by Michael Rodans, page 64, unknown, and appendix illustrations, by Margaret Guay.

We dedicate this book
with love and gratitude to our mothers:

Emma Lee Bunting Missel

Margaretta Lackey Babb

CONTENTS

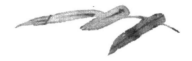

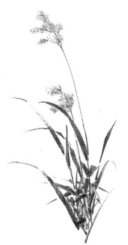

ACKNOWLEDGMENTS

Writing this book has presented us with many gifts and challenges; it has also required a discipline we never could have maintained without the indefatigable support of our families. We are deeply grateful to Libby's mother, Emma Lee Bunting Missel, for her enthusiastic and insightful gathering of relevant background data; Maggie's mother, Margaretta Babb, for her generous support; our fathers, James F. Bunting, Ph.D., and Dudley C. Babb, M.D., for teaching us to serve others and take care of ourselves; our husbands: Tom, for his background research, Don, for his proofreading, and both for their sense of humor and their willingness to do whatever needed to be done to hold home, office, and family together; our children: Deborah, David, Maria, Ben, Angus, and Sophie for their love and inspiration. Deborah for cooking nourishing, beautiful Ayurvedic meals; David for his sense of humor, encouragement, and participation with Maria in helping to create the inspiring Japanese Garden; Maria for unstintingly giving her summer to be nanny for her younger brother and sister and to read and reread the manuscript, gently challenging us to be clear; Ben for his humor, suggestions, and computer expertise; Angus and Sophie, whose understanding and tolerance beyond their years made it possible for us to stay focused. We offer profound thanks to Tom, Deborah, Ben, and Dorothy Meinhold for their heroic help in the office. We are grateful to Buff for letting Maggie in and training her.

We acknowledge the lineage of the Reiki grand masters: Mikao Usui, Chujiro Hayashi, and Hawayo Takata as well as the current lineage bearer, Phyllis Lei Furumoto, and the current head of the discipline, Paul David Mitchell. Hawayo Takata trained Barbara Lincoln McCullough as a Reiki master, who trained Judy-Carol Stewart, who trained Libby, who trained Maggie. We also wish to acknowledge all the masters of The Reiki Alliance who live the commitment to steward the Usui System of Reiki Healing.

Heartfelt thanks to Pamela Pettinati, M.D., who generously contributed her medical wisdom to the manuscript and assisted with proofreading and copyediting; Dick Nevell and Susan Bartlett for their advice and encouragement, which helped us clarify our ideas and direction in the beginning phases; Jim Powers, D.C., for his abiding care and wisdom; Donna Sherry, P.C., for her humor, brilliance, and wise guidance; Dom and Cindy DiSalvo for their generous offering of the writers' five-star haven; Jane Miller for her daily nurturing; Joyce Pereira and Coen Gootjes for their transformational Open Course; Susanne Robinson for her caring and coaching in integrating the Open principles into the Reiki Resolution Technique; Jo Barginear for her clarity and insight; Erica Baern and Nancy Stillman for their ongoing support and sense of humor; Marie Shanahan, R.N., Joyce Gale, R.N., Melissa Nelson, R.N., Don Catino, M.D., Lisa Olson, Calla Wells, MSW, M.Ed., Bettina Peyton, M.D., Cheryl Sterling, and Carroll French for their enthusiastic demonstrations of Reiki in action. We especially acknowledge the writing expertise of Susan Davidson, our editor; the artistic talent of Margaret Guay, the appendix illustrator, and the vision and perseverance of Robin Dutcher-Bayer, acquisitions editor, who started it all.

We express deep appreciation to all of our Reiki students, clients, and Reiki master candidates who chose us to be their teachers and from whom we have learned so much. Your genuine caring has inspired and fueled us over the years. We extend warm thanks to all of you who have so lovingly contributed support and stories to this book. It is our utmost joy and privilege to share this ancient, sacred form of healing with you.

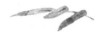

PREFACE:
OUR ORIGINS

Libby: I was instilled from childhood with my parent's YMCA philosophy of enhancing the health of the individual's body, mind, and spirit to effect world peace and understanding. This prepared me for a career of service. I trained at the Simmons College School of Social Work and became a medical social worker at Massachusetts General Hospital. Although I loved my work, I often longed to have something more to offer patients to take home with them to augment their healing process. In time I began to reflect on what preventive measures might be available that I could present to clients to support their well-being.

I first heard about Reiki when a friend from our Waldorf school invited me to a class. Even though I had never heard of Reiki, something prompted me to go. At the time, my two children were five and two years old, and I thought it might be helpful with the typical cuts and bruises of childhood. During class I worried that I might not be able to do Reiki, since I had no idea what energy healing was. My Reiki teacher, John Harvey Gray, assured me, however, that Reiki's effectiveness did not depend on my under-standing of it.

I began using Reiki on myself, the children, my husband, and our dog to help with injuries and upsets. Reiki became a reliable comfort for all of us. It really caught my attention when nurses told me my son's broken wrist had healed in two-thirds the expected time. After seeing the difference Reiki made in our family life, I was curious to know how it might facilitate therapy with clients. I chose to introduce Reiki to a client who was in a cast because of a ruptured Achilles tendon. Reiki not only supported his physical healing, but also enabled him to gain deeper clarity and insight regarding long-standing emotional issues, allowing him to come to new resolutions.

Following this successful inclusion of Reiki in the therapeutic process, I began incorporating it into my work with other clients when appropriate. As I watched Reiki accelerate the physical healing and spiritual growth of my clients, I realized that here was the something more I had wanted to give patients when at Massachusetts General Hospital. Now clients actively seek me out because they have heard that I combine Reiki with psychotherapy.

Maggie: My first experience of Reiki occurred when a dear friend gave me a Reiki treatment following the birth of my fourth child. Feeling exhausted after the exertion of childbirth, it was remarkable how blissful I became as my body eagerly pulled in the Reiki. My friend told me that I could learn it, and I was excited at the thought of being able to use Reiki with my husband and children. Reiki proved practical and useful with family life beyond expectation, but I was utterly surprised and delighted with the depth of its contribution to my personal life. It had a profoundly transformative effect.

With the help of Reiki I was able to choose new ways of being that invited balance, harmony, and wholeness into my life. I developed the confidence to say no to the things that were not supporting my growth and the strength to make decisions that I knew were correct for me. The more I dared to examine my beliefs and feelings and align them with what was true for me, the stronger my confidence and self-empowerment became. I experienced a dramatic blossoming and coming into my own. Gone was the victim role as I became more and more self-referred. Today Reiki continues to enhance every area of my life: embellishing my teaching skills, adding new creative impulse to my art, and deepening my spiritual development.

Libby and Maggie: When we met, ours was an instant connection. We recognized a common commitment to being increasingly open to the dynamic flow of universal life force in our lives to promote personal growth and evolution. Our similar values and vision for using Reiki to achieve full healing and optimal well-being for ourselves and others set the stage for working together. Out of our experience of teaching Reiki in mainstream health-care settings grew the inspiration and impetus for collaborating on this book to communicate the relevance of this ancient healing art to modern life. The vast array of accomplishments and healings of clients and students that we have been privileged to witness compel us to present our findings and understanding of Reiki for your consideration.

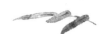

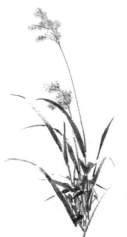

FOREWORD

*T*hese are times of great change. In the practice of medicine informational, technical, financial, relational, and spiritual forces are reshaping the way physicians and institutions administer to the patients in their care. As social and technological factors continue to impact the field of medicine, one element must never be lost. That element is the living relationship that health-care providers create with all those we care for—our patients, our community, and one another. These relationships are central to actualizing the paradigm of health care that integrates healing and community.

Relationship is the medium through which all communication flows, including the feelings and concerns, the hopes and fears of the patient. Likewise, relationship provides the means by which the practitioner can communicate caring and compassion. Relationship is itself an important therapeutic tool, one that often gets little formal acknowledgment.

More than fifty years ago Dr. Francis Peabody wrote in the *Journal of the American Medical Association* that "One of the essential qualities of the clinician is interest in humanity, for the secret of the care of the patient is caring for the patient."[1] It seems that somehow over the course of the past century this fundamental understanding has been lost. During that time, we have seen an explosive growth in modern, scientific biomedicine, occurring in a world where pneumonia, tuberculosis, polio, diptheria, smallpox, and other age-old diseases once were common, and shortened or compromised the lives of many people. As these conditions were successfully treated, health problems related to longevity, personal health habits, and lifestyle began to emerge. At the time of this writing, several leading causes of death, including heart disease, stroke, and cancer, are largely preventable by changing behaviors. However, due to a scientific paradigm that has traditionally applied surgical and pharmaceutical "solutions" to health problems, modern medicine has, to date, inadequately addressed lifestyle-related illnesses. Only recently have physicians begun to recognize that there are other important determinants of health.

The importance of relationship is beginning to be spoken about by some visionaries in the health-care field. And recent research findings have strongly suggested that psychosocial factors play a much more significant role in health than has ever been previously understood. Slowly it is being recognized that the way we think and feel—whether we feel cared for and nurtured and have a sense of meaning in life—have an effect on the course of disease. The implications of these findings on public health policy, medical practice, and medical education are profound. What if the quality of a physician's relationship with his or her patients affects health outcomes as much as our technical skills and interventions? An understanding of this connection would undoubtedly affect the way medicine is practiced and taught. This issue begs further research. Dr. Rachel Naomi Remen, Founder and Director of the Institute for the Study of Health and Illness, has written, "In short, the real question embedded in this research may be, 'Is there such a thing as a life-affirming relationship, and if so, what relationships are life-affirming and what relationships are not?' What we learn from asking this question may change the face of medicine."[2]

Health care as it is largely practiced today disregards the role of relationship in the healing process. In a field where technical competence is of greater value than interpersonal skills, our technical advances have far exceeded those of our predecessors, but our skills on the human level have not. This deficiency in psychosocial skills often leads to poor communication on the part of physicians who are unable or unwilling to discuss issues that are important to the patient, or to take the time to simply listen. As the dispensing of health care is relegated to a system of managers and "gatekeepers," do we risk losing forever the sense of purpose, the sense of meaning, that is the very essence of health care? After all, healing is a basic human activity, given meaning by people in relationship with one another and with community.

To understand the risk of the loss of caring relationship to our collective health and well-being, we must look deeper than the current debates over health-care reform and finance, or even the high-tech versus high-touch dialogues. Dr. Larry Dossey writes:

> At the root of the problem lies the fact that we, as a culture, have turned our collective back on healing. We should not kid ourselves: we are all in this together, jointly entranced by a physicalistic approach to health and illness, and dazzled by the promises of technology to right every conceivable misfire of the body. Against this backdrop, healers and healing have been shoved aside and very nearly forgotten, and we are paying the price. Ignoring the role of consciousness, soul, spirit, and meaning . . . we have birthed a malaise that permeates not just healers and healing, but the soul and the spirit of a culture.[3]

Fortunately there are positive changes occurring in health care that can help set us back on a healing path. This book is about one of those changes. *Reiki Energy Medicine* is not a book about techniques. Rather, it is a story of intention and an illumination of the work of its authors, who have chosen to enter into a different kind of relationship with those they care for. Reiki is about a return to relationship. In this book, Libby Barnett and Maggie Chambers show us one path that has brought healing to the lives of many people and give us a model for integrating complementary practices with the mainstream of health care. The authors offer the wisdom of Reiki not as an absolute answer, but as a choice that many health-care professionals have found to be a beneficial adjunct in their encounters with illness, pain, and suffering.

Reiki Energy Medicine is a guide for approaching all healing work with the intention that it serve the highest good—that it serve and affirm life. The authors show us how to awaken to a different way of being as healers, tempering scientific knowledge with wisdom and undertaking all actions under the guidance of compassion and love. Through these portals, the healing relationship is formed and found again.

ROBERT M. RUFSVOLD, M.D.
President and Medical Director
Wellspring Foundation of New England
and the Wellspring Cancer Help Program
Lyme, New Hampshire

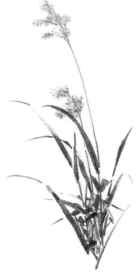

Chapter 1

UNIVERSAL LIFE FORCE: THE FUNDAMENTAL PRINCIPLE OF HEALTH

*A*n invisible but palpable life-force energy infuses and permeates all living forms. This energy is infinite, limitless, and pure. Intangible, it constantly bathes us. Inaudible and invisible, it fills us with peace. Odorless and tasteless, it sustains us. Although we swim in it, ingesting it with every breath, we are often unaware of its existence. Every living thing lives inside of and is inspirited by this force field.

This life-force energy is the essence that gives vitality to form. It is the primary activating energy of life and the underlying creative intelligence of the universe that organizes our world and everything in it. Ancient civilizations understood that this life-force energy flowed through the body, supporting optimal development and fulfillment. The Chinese identified this energy as *chi* (pronounced *chee*), the Indians called it *prana,* and the Japanese knew it as *ki.*

Because our culture has separated science from philosophy, based on the Cartesian separation of mind, body, and spirit, the concept of such a subtle yet powerful life-force energy has so far existed outside the theoretical framework of modern Western medicine. It is, therefore, challenging to discuss either the nature or the source of *chi, prana,* or *ki* in specific terms, since we do not even have an equivalent word for this energy in our culture. In a few studies, attempts have been made to measure this energy in the knowledge that quantifying it will validate this energetic phenomenon to the vast majority in the Western world who value objective test results over subjective experience. While this life-force energy resists quantifying, it is nevertheless pervasive; it exists within and all around us, deeply affecting our bodies, minds, and emotions. The ancients understood life-force energy to be in perfect balance in the body when a person experienced physiological orderliness, psychological equilibrium, and emotional stability.

Reiki (pronounced **ray**-*key*) is a precise method for connecting this universal energy with the body's innate powers of healing. Rediscovered in the mid-1800s by Dr. Mikao Usui, a Japanese monk educator, Reiki's origins are found in the Tibetan sutras, ancient records of cosmology and philosophy. This hands-on healing art, a powerful adjunct to conventional therapeutic modalities, fuels the body's homeostatic mechanisms and thereby assists in the restoration of balance on the physical, mental, and emotional levels. Because this life-force energy supports optimal development and fulfillment, Reiki promotes the highest healing good for all living things.

The biological intelligence that marshals the body's resources to heal a cut finger, mend a broken bone, help the lungs to breathe, or ease the transition into death is amplified by Reiki. Thus, as a healing modality it fits perfectly into the new paradigm of health emerging in Western medicine, a paradigm that includes mind/body awareness and prevention techniques. Over the past seven years we have taught Reiki to physicians, nurses, psychologists, psychotherapists, ministers, priests, nuns, physical and occupational therapists, hospice staff, and others. Some health-care organizations that are beginning to investigate complementary therapies have endorsed Reiki as a valuable part of the ongoing education for their professional staff. The following is a list of some of the institutions that either have invited us to teach an in-service Reiki program or have sent staff to us for training, often paying their tuition: The Harvard Community Health Plan; the Medical Center of Central Massachusetts; Cedarcrest Residential Center for Handicapped Children; Concord Regional VNA-Hospice House; Wentworth-Douglass Hospital, Dover, NH; Androscoggin Home Health Services, Lewiston, ME; Englewood Hospital and Medical Center, Englewood, NJ; VNA of the Greater Milford/Nothbridge Area, Mendon, MA; Emerson Hospital, Concord, MA; Healthcare Therapy Services, Indianapolis, IN; New London Hospital, NH; and Southern New Hampshire Medical Center. In a Reiki class, health-care professionals learn a method to augment their medical skills while also receiving an invaluable tool for attending to their own health maintenance, self-renewal, and personal growth.

The essential vehicle of Reiki is touch applied wherever and whenever appropriate. Because the practice of Reiki does not require complicated techniques, practitioners of many and varied disciplines are able to incorporate it easily into their specialties. By virtue of the fact that it enhances their healing skills and is also a rejuvenating practice of self-care, Reiki is becoming an important bridge of communication among a wide range of health-care providers.

In the near absence of scientific data to prove its effectiveness, theory and philosophy can help create a context for the mind to grasp the concept of Reiki. The best way to know that Reiki works, however, is to experience it. During Reiki treatment (see Appendix I and II) some people feel deep relaxation whereas others feel subtle sensations. Some people feel nothing at all. Regardless of the immediate impression, however, Reiki always acts upon the recipient even when its effects are not immediately perceptible. Results are not always evident during a Reiki session; for some people the healing shifts occur over time, while for others the changes are immediate and lasting.

Jack came to a Reiki clinic and received a session; his experience was one of mild relaxation. One year later Jack called full of anxiety because he had just been diagnosed with a hernia that required surgery. "I can't afford this. I don't have any insurance. My brother and father had hernias, and my brother had a long, painful recuperation. I'm self-employed; I can't afford to lose time. Will Reiki fix this?" We told Jack that we can never predict the results of Reiki, but Reiki sessions would be valuable because the inflow of life energy would help prepare him for surgery and aid his recuperation. As it is ideal to have a series of Reiki treatments for any serious condition, we arranged dates for four sessions. Then we suggested that Jack consider taking a class so he could do Reiki on himself between sessions.

Jack chose to take a Reiki class. At the end of the weekend he summed up his experience by saying, "It was nice, but it was very subtle." Two days later Jack left a message cancelling his four appointments. We imagined that because his physical experience during class was not strong and palpable, Jack had decided not to give Reiki a further chance to help heal his hernia. Later he told us that he had canceled his appointments because he could no longer find the hernia. We encouraged him to keep his appointment with his doctor to verify that he did not need the surgery and to have his healing documented. The physician verified that Jack's hernia was gone.

Through inducing the relaxation response, Reiki encourages enhanced integrated functioning of the body's healing systems. Studies show that a deep state of relaxation acts through the autonomic nervous system to lower blood pressure and heart rate and to relieve tension and anxiety. This state of relaxation also augments the abilities of the immune system to defend against bacteria and viruses, and it stimulates the brain's production of endorphins, natural opiates that act to decrease the perception of pain and create a state of well-being. The stimulation of this response through Reiki treatment, coupled with the increased and unimpeded flow of life-force energy through the body, encourages healing at all levels.

Reiki supports the recipient in taking charge of his process, acknowledging that the one receiving the treatment holds the power to heal. By its very nature Reiki gives the power and control for healing to the receiver, where it rightly belongs. The

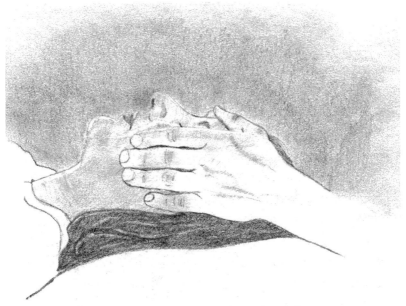

Reiki gives the power and control for healing to the receiver

inherent intelligence of the receiver's body knows what is needed and directs the life force to the highest priority. Whether by the mobilization of red blood cells to correct anemia, the knitting of bone to heal a fracture, the energy to complete a painstaking project, the clarity to resolve a conflict, or the inspiration to contact a friend long out of touch, the universal energy acts upon the recipient in a way that is most consonant with that person's highest healing good at that given moment in time.

With Reiki there is no body manipulation, only physical touch inspirited by universal life energy. Appropriate, safe touch in and of itself is very soothing and relaxing. Reiki combines the healing power of touch with life-force energy, made available to the student through a series of initiations that serve to balance and fine-tune the student's personal energy fields. (These fields will be discussed in chapter 2.) The four initiations are given by a Reiki master, connecting those who receive them to the lineage of Dr. Usui. Once you have been initiated, universal life energy is consistently available to you, because the initiation raises the frequency of the vibratory rate of your personal energy field to a higher level: a level where healing can occur at every moment. You become proficient at doing Reiki on yourself and others, thus freeing yourself from having to rely on someone else in order to receive the benefits of a Reiki session. Not just for repair or treating illness, Reiki provides you with a complete system for self-healing and optimal wellness that you can immediately implement in your daily life.

With the raising of consciousness in the West, Reiki is growing in popularity; more and more people are becoming aware of it and are using it. In 1971, when Libby was working at Boston's Massachusetts General Hospital as a social worker in pediatrics and child psychology, neither she nor any of her colleagues discussed energy healing. By contrast, in 1995 the Mind-Body

Medicine Group at Massachusetts General Hospital sponsored a conference to which Libby and other Reiki practitioners were invited to present Reiki. This event was well attended by over 300 employees, patients, and families of patients as well as by the general public. During the conference one of the coordinators asked Libby and a colleague to give Reiki treatments to hospitalized cancer patients who had requested them. Libby recalls, "It was gratifying to take Reiki where it was so appreciated and to watch it bring comfort in a very short time. We spent about fifteen minutes with each patient, putting our hands where we could comfortably touch the patient without disturbing any of the surrounding medical equipment. When family members were present, we often did Reiki on them as well. Tension and anguish were visibly alleviated. The patient felt better, the family felt better, and the staff was grateful for the support Reiki provided." After witnessing the effects of Reiki on their patients, some of the nurses went downstairs to the conference to receive a half-hour Reiki treatment for themselves. A few weeks later one of the coordinators of the conference came to class to learn Reiki.

REIKI AND THE MEDICAL REVOLUTION

The standard Western medical model pays far more attention to what constitutes disease than to what contributes to health. Allopathic medicine has historically tended to view disease as incorrect physical functioning caused primarily by infection, diet, environment, or heredity and to respond by planning a strategy of attack. While disease may at times arise in the physical body as an identifiable illness such as cancer, lupus, or arteriosclerosis, at other times it manifests in our mental or emotional bodies as states of dis-ease such as anxiety, depression, or paranoia. Disease can be more broadly defined, therefore, as a state of imbalance that causes disruption in optimal functioning of the body, mind, and emotions. Disease is not separate from the body; it is the body out of balance. Rather than being seen as an invader to be attacked and conquered, disease can be understood as an important messenger carrying the word that homeostasis needs to be restored.

Healing involves moving toward wholeness. Healing gently dissolves limiting thoughts and moves us toward acceptance of all aspects of ourselves. This is a state of living with awareness, in balance and harmony with ourselves and our environment and with the intention of expressing ourselves authentically in all areas of life. In this state of awareness we experience humor, vitality, organization, self-acceptance, creativity, flexibility, intuitive understanding, and clarity of thought. This is optimal well-being.

When we view the human being as a dynamic energy system, we realize that health is not a static goal. As current research suggests that the world we see is more than just matter, and the body is more than just a collection of functioning parts, there is increased curiosity about subtle energy and the role it plays in healing. With increasing interest in the mind's influence on bodily health, credible medical experts such as Herbert Benson, Joan Borysenko, Deepak Chopra, Barbara and Larry Dossey, David Eisenberg, Richard Gerber, Jon Kabat-Zinn, Ted Kaptchuk, Christiane Northrup, Mehmet Oz, Bernie Siegel, and Andrew Weil are leading the efforts to articulate a new way of viewing the mind/body relationship. Alternative medicine, a topic once confined to health-food stores and new-age venues, is now the subject of television and radio shows and books on the best-seller lists. In the five-part PBS series "Healing and the Mind," Bill Moyers reviews China's ancient medical traditions wherein therapists refer to the mysterious mental/physical energy known as *chi,* which pervades both mind and body and is the basis for good health. Moyers presents convincing evidence that the link between body and mind is intimate and profound. Deepak Chopra reflects this in his book *Ageless Body, Timeless Mind* when he states, "Our cells are constantly eavesdropping on our thoughts and being changed by them."[1]

In 1992 the National Institutes of Health established the Office of Alternative Medicine under pressure from a Congress alarmed by the soaring costs of health care and the frustrating fact that so many ailments—including AIDS, cancer, arthritis, back pain, arteriosclerosis, and heart disease—have yet to yield to standard medical interventions. In the interim a hungry public, desperate to have its health concerns met in ways that feel most promising of healthful resolution, is searching for alternatives without waiting for research to endorse personal choices. Americans have turned with growing enthusiasm to an array of complementary healing modalities. According to the *New England Journal of Medicine,* in 1990 one-third of the population of the United States consulted health-care providers other than conventional medical doctors, spending nearly fourteen billion dollars for their services, three-quarters of which was spent out-of-pocket.[2] The proliferation of healers practicing alternative forms of therapy, and the clients supporting their work, suggest that this trend continues to escalate.

In the intensifying search to find a solution to the high cost of medical care, complementary methods are slowly becoming recognized as important because they are cost-effective and they work. Reaching out to explore the field of mind/body healing in order to improve the quality of patient care and simultaneously lower their costs, several hospitals and hospice organizations have invited us to teach Reiki to their staffs. We appreciate the program directors' openness and willingness to go beyond their allopathic paradigm in order to experience Reiki and see how it might support their program goals.

At Dartmouth-Hitchcock Medical Center in New Hampshire, the Office of Continuing Education in the Health Sciences and the Hematology-Oncology Unit cosponsored a Reiki class for registered nurses and other health-care professionals in New England. Many of the nurses and physicians in attendance expressed concern that, in spite of their deep commitment to their work, something was missing from their interactions with their patients. Reiki supplied these health-care providers with the missing element. At the end of class they realized that not only did they have a powerful and effective new tool for encouraging homeostasis and promoting compassionate connection—both of

Colleagues can offer Reiki in brief, informal encounters

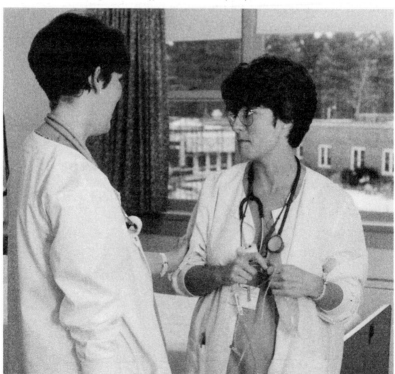

which would enhance their professional skills—but also they had an invaluable vehicle for achieving and maintaining personal well-being. For several of those present, this Reiki class was a benchmark experience in recognizing the importance and necessity of taking care of themselves. The high enrollment and the overwhelmingly positive feedback on the evaluations prompted the administration to offer the program again, and it was equally well received the second time.

At the Medical Center of Central Massachusetts the anesthesiology staff had witnessed how hypnotherapy and therapeutic touch helped to shorten the length of time that patients spent in the postanesthesia care unit (the recovery room), as well as the length of their total hospital stay. These nurses came to Reiki class because they were eager to find additional mind/body modalities to expand their professional skills. When medical professionals integrate Reiki routinely with their regular procedures, patients often report feeling less pain and anxiety, require fewer medications, and have quicker recovery times.

In the 1990s we have entered the age of energy information. Because we live in a constantly expanding world with continually changing paradigms, it is imperative that we maintain flexibility in order to stay aware of and involved with this ever-changing world. Our evolution now depends upon teaming the analytical mind with sensate awareness. Daily, even moment by moment, we can choose how to respond to the abundance of new information continually being made available to us. Just as germs existed before the microscope was invented, subtle energy is a reality even though we cannot yet objectify it. It took Johns Hopkins Hospital ten years after the time that Joseph Lister first presented his findings on bacteria to begin using rubber gloves during surgical procedures. We each have a choice to be as innovative as Lister or as resistant as his colleagues. As we observe the effects of healing in the human energy field, health-care providers of all modalities have the opportunity to be part of the new vanguard in medicine, uniting mind and body in the efforts to promote holistic and cost-effective wellness. Reiki is a significant element in this important effort.

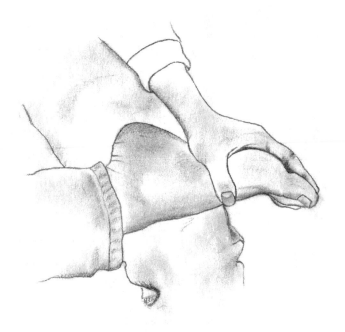

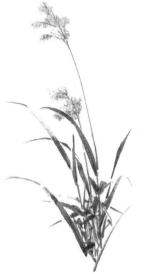

Chapter 2

THE UNIQUE
POWER OF REIKI

*I*n our culture we are conditioned to learn new information at an intellectual level first, and then to apply that conceptual knowing in such a way that it either supports or invalidates our firsthand experiences. This need for the mind to know creates an interesting challenge in teaching Reiki. Like a computer conducting a file search, the brain tries to link new information with something that it already understands. Because the concept of universal life energy is unfamiliar to most Westerners, the efforts of a new student to link energy healing with something already known proves impossible—the brain either becomes confused or inaccurately hooks up the concept of Reiki with something that Reiki is not. To deal with this dilemma, we speak in metaphors, analogies, and stories when we discuss Reiki and its effects, so that the mind can begin to understand what Reiki is.

Quantum physicists are developing new theories of energy movement and transformation that challenge traditional explanations of the nature of the universe. Their fascinating conjectures are slowly shifting the collective mind toward a new way of understanding our physical world, including the physical matter of our human bodies. Since energy healing is inexplicable within the confines of the mechanical model of the universe—the working model for the past four centuries, at least—we encourage students to be patient with themselves as they try to integrate their experiences of Reiki. Messages from the body can be easily overlooked when the brain is busy analyzing. Just because a person's conscious awareness is not attuned to the activity of peptides, receptors, and cells, however, does not make the existence of these biophysical phenomena any less crucial to the smooth functioning of the body. Similarly, our inability to explain in precise terms how the flow of universal life force throughout the body acts to maintain health does not make universal life energy invalid. We suggest, therefore, that students shift their focus from analyzing Reiki to observing their bodily-felt experiences, recognizing that much value can be obtained from noticing rather than analyzing it. Since the way of knowing that is supported by our culture rests on the supremacy of data, sensations that cannot be quantified are not considered viable information in determining the efficacy of a therapeutic procedure. As a society, we do not value sensation as a primary mode of perception. Yet, experience is sensation, and our bodily experiences cannot be denied.

When people continued to ask endless questions about Reiki from an intellectual standpoint, Hawayo Takata, one of the Reiki grand masters in the Usui lineage, would end the discussion by saying, "Just do Reiki! Do Reiki! Do Reiki!" She knew that the experience of channeling the universal life energy would lead people ultimately to an embodied understanding of the power of this ancient healing practice.

We choose our own attitude in approaching any new experience. When we choose to be influenced by limiting beliefs, we cheat ourselves out of having an authentic experience in that moment. If the mind decides that something is not worth considering, we may lose the chance to grow and expand. We invite our Reiki students to be democratic in their senses and to notice their experiences without judging, comparing, or needing to know precisely how the experience has been evoked. This way of engaging with their Reiki experiences is a way of being in beginner's mind: a willingness to stay open to all possibilities without needing to have all the answers.

When students are trying to understand Reiki, the familiar questions that arise are "What is Reiki?" and "What can it do?" These are the questions asked by many at the classes we teach at health care institutions and agencies. Students in these classes become filled with their Reiki experiences, and their minds are quieted. Feeling the sensations of life energy flowing through their hands and into themselves and their colleagues, the participants are less driven by the need to understand. Even though they cannot measure or otherwise quantify what is happening, neither can they deny their tangible, sensate experiences.

In working on the energetic plane, as we do with Reiki, the shifts and changes that take place for the receiver often happen at a nonmaterial level and therefore may be difficult to perceive. Nevertheless, healing is taking place for the recipient according to the highest priority in the holistic ordering of the universe. The effects of a Reiki session may be felt physically, or they may result in an attitude shift, a creative insight, a solution to a vexing problem, or in a host of other nonphysical ways. The proof of whether a therapeutic procedure is effective rests not on the gathering of data alone but on the client's actual experience— physical, mental, and emotional.

Because its nature and mode of action are not yet quantifiable, Reiki energy medicine is not easily evaluated by our current allopathic medical and clinical protocols. Historically allopathic medicine has dismissed anomalous events outside its framework of healing, one that is based on structure and function relationships. Since the effects that seem to be stimulated or quickened by Reiki are often considered unusual from a conventional medical point of view, Reiki falls into the category of the inexplicable. The Office of Alternative Medicine is funding grants to evaluate the efficacy of complementary therapies. If Reiki is to be seriously investigated, current research methodologies need to be expanded in order to accurately measure Reiki's impact on outcomes. Until sufficient research on the effects of Reiki is funded and conducted, we must depend on anecdotal evidence to create the possibility in peoples' minds that Reiki does, in fact, work.

One of the first attempts to document the effects of Reiki was conducted by Wendy Wetzel, R.N., as part of her master's thesis at Sonoma State University. The study states that "In subjects receiving First Degree Reiki training, there was a significant change in the oxygen-carrying capability [of blood] within a twenty-four-hour period [following initiation] as reflected by measurement of hemoglobin and hematocrit values, significant at the P=.01 levels." The study concludes that "Reiki seems a natural adjunct to nursing care. . . . Reiki could be integrated into every area of nursing practice. . . . It connects us as nurses to a Universal Force. . . . It can reduce the experience of burnout and job-related stress. It is an agent to nurture the nurse."[1]

Now that Reiki is gaining in popularity and exposure, it is just a matter of time before we have more facts to satisfy the intellect. Larry Dossey, M.D., author of *Healing Words: The Power of Prayer and the Practice of Medicine,* explains that although extensive research is now being done on the power of prayer to help ease the pain of terminal conditions or affect the outcome of surgical procedures, people are not withholding prayer or meditation as they wait for further research results to validate the efficacy of these actions. Like prayer, Reiki is a modality that cannot yet be fully explained but nevertheless has been demonstrated time and again to be an important complement to allopathic procedures.

Once students have begun to practice Reiki during class, the feeling of universal life energy flowing through them creates an experiential bridge to the mind, providing them with something to hold onto until they accumulate enough experiences to ground them in the certainty that Reiki works. From their personal experiences, and through hearing our many anecdotes, our students are able to create a new framework of thought that includes Reiki.

Eight-year-old Bobby received a crushed skull and massive internal bleeding from a skiing accident. He was transported by helicopter from a local hospital emergency room to a larger city hospital. Bobby's mother, Mary, who already knew how to do Reiki, was able to have her hands on Bobby during the helicopter flight. She stayed out of the way of the emergency medical team, placing her hands on Bobby's feet and lower legs. She also put her hands on herself, using Reiki to calm her own fears. A nurse later told Libby that as the helicopter took off, the pilot reported, "They don't think he's going to make it." Libby joined Mary and Bobby in the emergency room.

Mary and Libby stood quietly next to the gurney with their hands on Bobby, giving him Reiki between diagnostic procedures. The staff welcomed their participation and were pleased that Bobby was not left alone when they had to attend to other patients.

Bobby required eight hours of surgery to reconstruct his skull. To decrease their anxieties, Mary and Libby gave Reiki to themselves and to each other while they waited for the surgery to be completed. Following surgery, Libby and Mary were invited into the intensive care unit by the hospital staff, where they continued to do Reiki on Bobby. The staff fully accepted Mary and Libby putting their hands on Bobby. Some of the physicians and nurses had heard about Reiki and asked questions about it. They knew the comforting value of touch and were open to the possibility that Reiki might assist Bobby's healing process. Clearly it was not hurting, and if it made him feel better, they were in favor of it.

Mary and Libby continued to practice Reiki on Bobby during his three-week hospital stay. The staff grew increasingly enthusiastic about Reiki as they repeatedly witnessed how it calmed Bobby and eased his pain. During Bobby's recuperation at home, Mary continued to use Reiki on Bobby for the loving connection and support it provided. Although seizures are very common with this type of head injury, Bobby had none. Moreover, he recovered sooner than had been predicted. He had no residual impairment and was able to resume his normal activities within two months.

This anecdote demonstrates how Reiki can effectively blend with conventional medicine. Recovery from such a traumatic injury as Bobby's requires deep, extensive healing. While the surgeon's expertise was essential, the excellent nursing care and the loving attention of family and friends all supported Bobby in his healing process. The part Reiki may have played in Bobby's recovery cannot yet be documented by standard research methods. However, Reiki was one of the consistent components of Bobby's care plan, and subjective feedback suggests that Reiki made a difference in his comfort and well-being.

Bobby's is one of the countless experiences in which the presence of Reiki seems to have assisted and accelerated a complicated healing process. With its impulse toward balance and wholeness, Reiki is a powerful adjunct to medical intervention

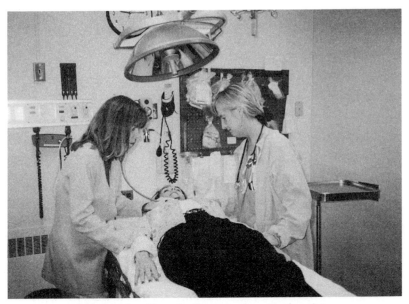

Reiki blends with and enhances conventional medicine

and care. As Pamela Pettinati, M.D., a reconstructive surgeon at Saint Elizabeth's Medical Center in Boston, states, "Reiki helps the patient feel better and heal better." In our classes we share many stories like Bobby's. Theories can be debated forever from different points of view, but when you have an experience of something working, the debate becomes irrelevant. One surgeon we have trained reports that she is often called upon to perform Reiki as a last resort when the conventional medical procedures do not appear to be sufficient. While her colleagues may not understand Reiki, they see that it works and they value the results.

THE HUMAN ENERGY SYSTEM

Modern physics is now discovering what the ancients knew—that our bodies are not solid entities but rather are interacting fields of energy given to continuous, creative fluctuation. From the smallest subatomic particles to the space beyond the skin to the farthest reaches of the universe, vibratory forces configure

19

and reconfigure who we are in ourselves, in our relationships, and in the world. Quantum physics has demonstrated that all substance is composed of energy fields: vast expanses of space in which particles of matter are created by the temporary intersection of these fields of energy.

While fairly new to Westerners, this concept is deeply rooted in the thought and writings of Eastern cultures. In ancient India, China, Japan, and Egypt it was understood that the human body is made up of dynamic energy systems. Even though we cannot see these energy systems that compose and sustain the body/mind, they are nevertheless a vital part of us. These energy fields interact not only within the individual but also between individuals and within the environment. The more we are able to sense and understand ourselves as fields of energy rather than solid, particulate structures, the better able we are to understand the mind/body connection and how it affects our quality of life.

The chakra-nadi system and the acupuncture meridian system are two ancient models that describe the flow of universal life-force energy within the body. The chakra-nadi model is thought to have originated in India; the acupuncture meridian model is attributed to the Chinese.

Chakras, Sanskrit for "wheels," are nonphysical vortices of energy that transmute vital life force into forms usable for the functioning of the body and mind. The chakras are connected to each other and the physical body through the *nadis:* energetic threads through which universal life energy flows. The seven major chakras are located parallel to the spine, from the area of the coccyx (the tailbone) to the top of the head. They correspond to the endocrine glands and the six major nerve plexuses of the body. Primarily responsible for the chemical homeostasis of the body, the endocrine system works to balance the body's physical energy and stabilize mental and emotional functioning.

20

The nerve plexuses, points of confluence within the nervous system, influence greatly one's patterns of activity and rest.

In the Chinese system of energy healing, the *acupuncture points* are energetic doorways in the skin through which vital life energy flows from the universal field into the human energy field and physical body. The *meridians* are a system of conduits through which *chi* flows throughout the body to the nerves, blood vessels, and organs. Richard Gerber, M.D., author of *Vibrational Medicine,* acknowledges a relationship between these two models when he says, "Although the digestive system takes in biochemical energy and molecular building blocks in the form of physical nutrients, the chakras, in conjunction with the acupuncture meridian system, take in higher vibrational energies that are just as integral to the proper growth and maintenance of physical life."[2]

The physical body is the most dense and therefore the most familiar aspect of the human energy system. Extending beyond the physical body are multiple subtle bodies through which vital energy flows from the universe into the physical being. These energy fields interpenetrate each other and the physical body, and thus have a very powerful effect on our well-being, directly influencing the condition of our physical, mental, and emotional health. Though not composed of matter, the subtle bodies are perceptible through touch and are often experienced by Reiki students as well as by practitioners of other ancient systems of medicine, such as Ayurveda and acupuncture. Energy manifests as substance, and so it is that specific energetic patterns can be expressed as illness or lack of ease in the physical body. All conditions of imbalance are rooted in the human energy field, and it is the underlying energetic patterns that must be addressed and resolved in order to create conditions for wellness. This is the possibility offered by Reiki.

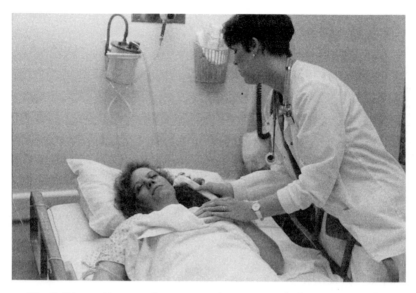

The Reiki practitioner conducts universal energy into the human energy field

The Reiki practitioner conducts vital energy from the universal energy field into the human energy field, where the energy is transmuted into a form that is usable at the cellular level. The vital energy recharges, realigns, and rebalances the subtle bodies, bringing harmony and wholeness to all the recipient's systems.

Unlike other forms of energy medicine, Reiki does not involve diagnosing imbalance in the recipient's energy field or intentionally repatterning the system. There is no possibility of misdiagnosis or energy overload with Reiki, because in any session it is the client who is in charge, her cells drawing in the amount of energy needed to bring the mind/body back to homeostasis. This all happens beyond the conscious mind—the client does not need to exert effort to pull in the life-force energy. It happens independently of belief system, emotional state, or religious preference. The body's inner intelligence orchestrates the entire session in accordance with the creative intelligence of the universe.

Because the theories of quantum physics are not yet universally accepted, the concept of energy healing confounds many, and so we speak in metaphors when we describe the effect of Reiki on the body. To introduce the ideas of the new physics, and yet stay very literal in our descriptions, we characterize the Reiki process as the body's cells pulling in the universal life force. We like to compare this process of the cells to that of barnacles living on the rocks along the seacoast, opening when the waves come in to receive their nourishment and to relinquish their waste. Similarly, during a Reiki session the client's cells open to pull in the universal life energy. As the cells open, they release the energy of all that is old, outmoded, irrelevant—all they have held onto that works against that person's highest good. This process of opening and releasing mirrors the flow of the universe—a continual taking in and letting go—with the ultimate goal being the balancing and harmonizing of the entire system. When the body is in balance, it can heal itself.

Not only is healing in a Reiki session determined by the recipient, it happens on a priority basis; thus, the result may differ from what the client wants or expects. Healing always happens during a Reiki session, although the effects of the healing may not be immediately perceptible to the client or the practitioner. Frequently it is unyielding pain that brings people to try Reiki as a last resort. Often they are rewarded not only with relief from the pain but with some other shifts as well.

Marion's immediate issue was chronic pain in her right ankle due to a severe injury. Three months of physical therapy gave her a feeling of stability and strength in the ankle but did not resolve the pain. The pain and her vulnerability to frequent sprains left Marion no option but to walk with crutches. When Libby saw her she had been on crutches for six months and was in constant discomfort. Two orthopedic surgeons had suggested either long-term bracing of the ankle or surgical intervention (a Brostrom-type repair to reef the lateral tissues). The latter would result in her being in a cast for at least two months. It was the beginning of the holiday season, and Marion could not imagine being immobilized throughout Thanksgiving and Christmas while caring for two small children. She came for a Reiki session hoping to find an alternative solution to her painful condition. When she called for an appointment, she asked if Reiki could heal her ankle so that she wouldn't require surgery. Libby explained that while Reiki offers no guarantees, it might help with pain relief. Since Reiki is noninvasive and gentle, it certainly would not aggravate her condition.

At the completion of her first session, Marion reported feeling more relaxed and less anxious. The next day she called Libby to say, "There's still no change in my ankle, but last night I wrote the outline to a children's book that has been in my head for the last fifteen years." Marion's first experience with Reiki did not eliminate her need for crutches but instead seemed to influence her creativity, demonstrating that healing happens on a priority basis. Having repeatedly observed this phenomenon, we say that Reiki gives you what you need, which may not always coincide with what you think you want at the time.

During her second Reiki session, one week later, Marion noticed that the swelling in her ankle was reduced; she could see the shape of the bone for the first time in months. At her third weekly Reiki session Marion arrived without crutches. Walking no longer resulted in sprains, and her pain was significantly diminished. After her fourth session Marion's condition was so improved that she consulted her doctor and canceled her surgery. Marion decided to learn Reiki so that she could support her healing by doing Reiki on herself between appointments. She took a Reiki class on the day she had been sched-uled for surgery.

Following two more appointments, Marion was able to maintain her restored health by doing self-Reiki. Her Christmas card reported *how well her ankle had healed and described the ease with which she was able to walk up the hill when sledding with her children. Over the next two and one-half years, Marion's children, husband, and sister all learned Reiki, since they had witnessed the profound difference it had made in Marion's life.*

The Reiki process highlights the truth about healing: that the power and the responsibility for healing lie within the individual. The Reiki practitioner brings intention and commitment to the process, acting as a compassionate conduit for the universal life force, but the practitioner does not *do* the healing for the client. The healing happens as a result of the relationship between the receiver's energy field and the universal energy field, mediated through the cellular consciousness of the receiver. Reiki empowers the receiver to do the healing that needs to be done on all levels of being.

Reiki is not a panacea. It works to enhance and accelerate the normal healing processes of the body and the mind. Reiki is not constrained by lack of knowledge, imagination, or

Reiki empowers the receiver to do the healing that needs to be done

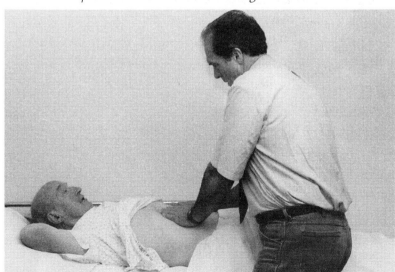

understanding. It is offered unconditionally and is received regardless of circumstance.

People are able to connect with the universal life energy in a variety of ways without the assistance of Reiki or other energy-based therapies. One way is through the food we eat. When we nourish ourselves with high-quality fresh foods that are lovingly prepared, we strengthen ourselves on all levels. There are also many ways we can be energized by the elements. When we are in physical contact with nature—outside in the sun, enjoying natural bodies of water and lush vegetation, climbing on rock, or feeling the wind embrace us—we are absorbing the vital life force always present and available to us. Such deep nourishment from nature relaxes and rejuvenates.

Meditation is another way people dip into life-force energy. The expanded state that can be achieved through meditation is one of pure awareness, true harmony, authentic self-power, and unity with all. Many meditators are unable, however, to sufficiently sustain their connection with this vital energy to bring peace, harmony, and wisdom into their daily lives on a consistent basis. In challenging situations it proves difficult to duplicate or maintain this connection with life-force energy. And though it sometimes happens that healing abilities are generated in a time of crisis, under less extreme circumstances the same abilities are usually not able to be called forth. For example, medical personnel often report responding to a severe emergency with skill far exceeding their usual expertise. Later, however, when the crisis has passed, they are unable to duplicate their performance. Reiki brings continuity to the process of connecting with universal life energy. Reiki gives individuals a consistent access into this energy. Whether one is involved with someone else's pain or emotional upheaval, or experiencing one's own distress, Reiki is immediately available.

THE REIKI INITIATION

Everyone is born with the capacity to heal. Most people, however, lack a form or structure for using this capacity, so they usually experience their innate healing resources in fleeting moments. The Reiki initiation empowers us to be instruments to assist the healing process whenever we put our hands on ourselves or another.

Performed by a traditionally trained Reiki master, the initiation is the key that enables us to access universal life energy easily and consistently. It is the initiation process that sets Reiki apart from other forms of hands-on energy work. In the Reiki class, four initiations raise the student's energy field to a higher vibratory level, activating fully the capacity to heal. Spending a brief time with each student, the Reiki master performs a sacred ceremony for each initiation based on the precise formula Dr. Usui rediscovered in the ancient Sanskrit texts. This ritual fine-tunes, balances, and aligns the student's energy system, empowering him to become a conduit for channeling universal life energy. Mrs. Takata compared the initiation process to a radio being tuned to a specific station. Like radio waves, universal life force is all around us. The initiation process "tunes" our energy fields so that we can receive the Reiki "frequency."

The initiations sensitize the student's hands, making them better able to conduct energy and detect energy flow. (Some practitioners liken their hands to electrodes.) Another result of the initiation is increased protection for dealing with environmental or situational circumstances, whether that be a crowded airport, an aggravating colleague, or a family member's emotional upset.

Experiences like the Reiki initiation that cannot be fully explained by the intellect can cause us to become so frustrated that we want to ignore or discredit them. For example, following the

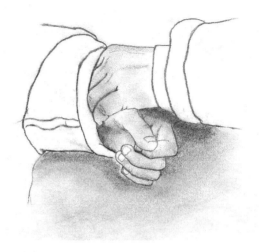

The initiations empower the student to conduct life force

initiations in a class we conducted at a hospital, numerous questions were raised as the healthcare professionals' minds grappled with how the initiations work. Even though they had heard that Reiki happens beyond the grasp of the intellect, there was a persistent desire among the students for a mental construct upon which to hang their initiation experiences. A physician finally spoke up, saying, "There is no need to know. We do not know how certain medications work, yet we prescribe them regularly because of their results." The same can be said of Reiki.

Though the initiation process is the same for everyone, the experience of it differs from person to person, demonstrating that the body's inner intelligence knows exactly what is needed for that person's highest healing good. Each person's inner wisdom creates the exact experience needed during the initiations, whether that is an answer, a vision, or an uplifting feeling providing the next step in the individual's personal healing journey.

For some the initiation is quiet and peaceful, while for others it is dramatic and intense. Many people see vivid colors and images; others see deities or the faces of loved ones. People often feel gently bathed in light or encircled by a fine sheath of energy. Frequently the experience is quite physical. A recovering addict experienced such deep satisfaction during initiation that his desire for drugs—a constant daily struggle—completely vanished and has not returned. A woman who had lived with a cloudiness in her eye for several years experienced a flash of bright light during her initiation. When she got home that night she realized that the cloudiness was gone and she could once again read fine print.

In 1967 Alex was in a very serious motorcycle accident that resulted in three crushed vertebrae. His doctors said it was likely that he would never walk again. However, with determination and perseverance Alex learned a specific pattern of muscle control that allowed him to walk, albeit with chronic pain. Alex's wife came to class to learn Reiki, hoping it would benefit her hospice volunteer work as well as provide some pain relief for her husband. She did Reiki on Alex immediately following class. He experienced such relief from his pain that he attended our next Reiki class. After his first initiation Alex sat wiggling his toes, looking incredulous. "Strange!" he exclaimed. "This is really strange. I have no pain! I can remember where the pain was—but now it's gone! I'm afraid to move. I'm afraid it will come back." For Alex the biggest challenge was to keep his mind from recreating the pain.

Alex remained pain free for two years. The following winter he fell on ice and broke his back again. Today Alex has a diagnosis of arthritis, spinal stenosis, and pinched nerves. Using self-Reiki throughout the day and receiving frequent one-half hour Reiki treatments from his wife enables Alex to manage his pain.

Often the shift that occurs during the initiations happens on a more subtle but clearly perceptible level. A physician at one of our classes was fascinated by a nurse's gradual change in attitude from analytical skepticism at the beginning of class to excited, enthusiastic confidence during practice time as she experienced the vital life force flowing through her hands. Witnessing this transformation, the physician was visibly moved. Three years later this nurse continues to regularly incorporate Reiki in care plans for the patients she sees as a visiting nurse. She is so enthusiastic about the results that she often refers colleagues to Reiki class.

The twenty-one days following the initiation are a time of heightened awareness for the Reiki graduate. Just as people have different experiences of the initiation, they have different experiences of this period of accelerated self-healing. For some this time is blissful; they experience an expansive love for everyone around them and feel a deep sense of oneness and connectedness with life. Others feel profoundly rejuvenated, as if they had gone through a cleansing or purification. The initiation tunes the subtle bodies to a higher vibratory level, aligning them more strongly with universal life force. As the aligned body is infused with this vital force, it is better able to cleanse itself. Negative thoughts and old conditioned behaviors of a lower vibration are not able to sustain themselves in the new energetic environment created by the initiation. They are released from the system, making room for increased intuition and creativity to be expressed on all levels.

Two weeks after class Terry called to report that the stress at work wasn't getting to him as much, and he was able to deal with people more easily. At the same time, he found himself naturally choosing foods that were better for him, so that some of the weight he had gained after he quit smoking was beginning to disappear.

Sometimes what happens following initiation is a delightful surprise, as one biological researcher from Massachusetts General Hospital discovered.

Frank called the day after class to tell us that he had received a severe blow to his head that morning. Spontaneously putting his hand on the injured spot, Frank said he wasn't even thinking about doing Reiki and yet he instantly felt liquid warmth flowing into the site and soothing his pain. His mind was critiquing the scenario in disbelief, knowing that the experience of intense warmth was happening faster than could be possible from a medical point of view. After the sensation of warmth subsided, there was no redness or swelling. Frank was astonished because, in his judgment, both symptoms should have been present, given the severity of the blow. Frank also reported with great delight that he and his wife, a pediatric dentist who had also attended class, felt like new lovers again.

As the initiations raise the vibrations of our energy bodies, vitality increases and old, dense patterns are released. It's not unusual for a new Reiki graduate to have a difficult emotional pattern simply drop away.

Joan went home after Reiki class to an all-too-familiar scene of her husband and son drinking heavily. As her son started to leave the house, Joan confronted him about endangering other people and took away his car keys. He was outraged, but she remained insistent. In Joan's words, "This was something I had longed to do but never dared. No longer was I going to put up with or feel responsible for his behavior."

Inherent in the Reiki initiation is the intention that healing always happen for the highest healing good. The flow of life-force energy is contingent upon intention as well as cellular demand; however, the energy flows without constant focus or verbal repetition of intention. This aspect of Reiki is particularly beneficial in emergency situations.

Intention to assist the healing process is implicit in the placing of our hands on our own body or another's. Many Reiki practitioners consciously employ intention and awareness of the

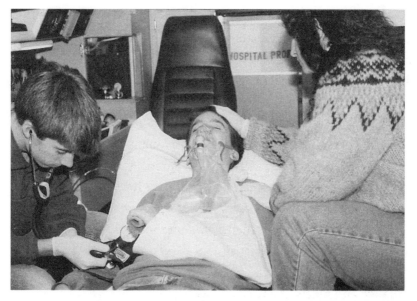

Reiki is particularly beneficial in emergency situations

flow of life energy as part of their practice. Following the Reiki
initiation, universal life energy flows through our hands in
response to our intention and the demand of the body's cells.
The flow is nothing we can will or force because it depends on
the cellular demand as directed by the recipient's innate intelligence, not on our ability to do. This means that whether the
practitioner places her hands on her patient, her child, a stranger,
or herself, the energetic flow is always available in response to
the cells' demand. Reiki's effectiveness does not depend on the
feelings or beliefs of either the practitioner or the recipient—
which is fortunate, given that beliefs and feelings are often what
limit, block, or challenge a healing process. The initiation goes
beyond our feelings and beliefs to connect both the practitioner
and the recipient with an unconditional and unlimited source of
life. This connection empowers us to channel universal life
energy for anyone, including ourselves. The energy is equally

available to the patient, the child, the stranger, or oneself because it is not contingent upon our intellectual conceptualization, our attitude, our agenda, or our mood.

Benefiting both client and practitioner, the performance of Reiki is a win-win situation. Contrary to what happens in many situations where we deplete ourselves in our efforts to help another, with Reiki we receive as we simultaneously give. Because we do not use our personal energy, there is no sacrificing of self for another. In fact, not only are we not depleted, we are energized as the vital energy flows through us. Many people comment that it doesn't matter whether they are giving or receiving Reiki; they experience a fullness of energy either way.

Our bodies are flowing energy systems that constantly change and renew themselves. Because they are continually reorganizing and restructuring, we have the opportunity in every moment to recreate ourselves toward a pattern of wholeness. Easily implemented, Reiki is a reliable tool for making universal life force available in order to mobilize our biological healing resources and accelerate our growth and development.

Throughout life we discover different tools to help us achieve our various objectives. In all of the therapeutic systems available today, there are few that speak unequivocally to our intrinsic hunger for wholeness. This yearning, felt throughout our society, motivates hundreds of thousands of people to seek therapy, find teachers, or read self-help books. The longing for a technique to support our human and personal evolution is summed up by noted scientist and energy healer Barbara Brennan in her book *Hands of Light*, when she says, "Perhaps someday we will be able to build a machine that can tap into the energy of the universal energy field and have all the energy we need without threat of harming ourselves."[3] This ability is Reiki. Someday is now.

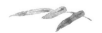

Chapter 3

SELF-REIKI: CARING FOR THE CAREGIVER

*M*ost people to whom we teach Reiki grew up with the directive to take care of others before taking care of themselves. This dictum demands that we make an effort to rest and rejuvenate only after we attend to all other responsibilities. The extra time or energy that might be devoted to self-caretaking has never been easy to find, in times past or in our modern day. As a result, many of us move frantically through our lives trying to finish everything on the "to do" list in order to have a moment for ourselves. When we live this way, propelled by this edict, those revitalizing moments are as elusive as a hummingbird, rarely alighting and gracing us with the presence of stillness. When we take care of everything and everyone else first, those treasured moments for true rejuvenation are seldom ever realized.

Those of us who work in the helping professions, caretakers by choice, are especially prone to disregarding our own needs in the service of others. Client appointments are always honored and met. Yet how

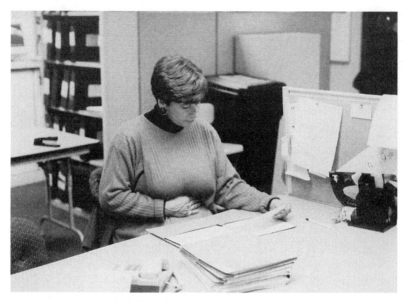

Reiki helps you regain clarity and perspective

many of us rigorously protect self-care time? Most of us regularly surrender it to the request of a client, a colleague, a family member, or a friend. Every massage therapist, for instance, knows the true ratio of massages given to massages received. Self-caretaking is something with which many people are unfamiliar, yet it is essential to living life in a state of balance and well-being. Taking care of oneself is not selfish, it is practical: an empty vessel has nothing to offer. If our desire is to help others, we must first be full within ourselves. Reiki is a way of achieving this fullness with little effort or time, yet the practice yields tremendous benefit for the caregiver. Reiki opens us to absorbing more of the vital life energy that ultimately directs and encourages all healing processes. This power helps us stay attuned and aligned within ourselves, keeping obstruction and exhaustion at a minimum and encouraging our healing resources to flow freely from within.

Self-Reiki is an effective method for centering yourself. If you find yourself feeling upset, angry, or afraid, a few minutes of

Reiki helps you feel calm, confident, and strong. When you are confused or overwhelmed by challenges, Reiki helps you regain clarity and perspective. When you feel pulled into the swamp of the mundane, you can extricate yourself with Reiki. It gets you through grueling days with tight schedules or long nights tending a sick patient. Self-Reiki allows you to build high levels of energy reserves for these challenging situations. By doing Reiki regularly on yourself, you are more resilient and resourceful in times of stress. Reiki helps you take care of yourself in order that you can take care of others.

THE REIKI SELF-TREATMENT PROTOCOL

A complete self-Reiki treatment comprises twelve to fifteen hand positions covering the front and back of the body. (The difference in number is due to the fact that some people add positions according to personal preference. See Appendix I.) The hands are placed gently but firmly on the body, remaining in each position for three to five minutes, or longer if desired. The

Reiki helps you through grueling days with tight schedules

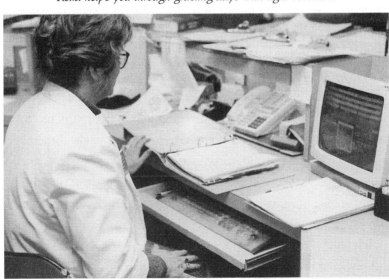

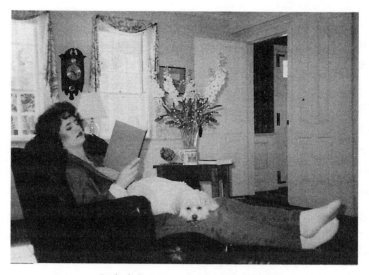

Reiki helps you take care of yourself

first position is at the top of the head; from there the hands move sequentially down the body, ending on the coccyx, at the base of the spine. Each position flows into the next in a relaxed, natural manner. Some people do not feel anything while giving themselves Reiki; others experience soothing, comforting sensations as they move through the different positions. When you put your Reiki-initiated hands on your body and then follow the form like a recipe, you are receiving nourishing, revitalizing life-force energy whether or not you register any sensations.

While the average time in each position in the traditional form is three to five minutes, you may choose to spend more time in any one position, depending on your need and your situation. For example, if you are experiencing tension in your abdomen, you may want to keep your hands there longer to provide the relief you need. How much time you allot to self-Reiki is an individual decision; it varies with how much time you choose to give yourself. Some people spend an average of twenty to forty minutes a day doing the self-Reiki treatment. A busy surgeon we taught combines self-Reiki with reading and contemplation time, increasing her total of time spent with herself to four hours daily.

Doing self-Reiki in the evening encourages you to drift into a deep, restful sleep. It is also a delightful way to bring yourself to wakefulness and prepare to meet the day with a fresh perspective. For some, implementing self-Reiki at the beginning or the end of each day becomes an important ritual, a time for reflection, relaxation, meditation, or prayer. Such nurturing ritual is largely missing from our contemporary lifestyles, and Reiki is one way to bring it back. I (Maggie) experience Reiki to be most profound when I take the time to give myself a complete self-treatment. I stretch out on my bed and slowly move through the positions as I contemplate the events of my day and the current issues in my life. Doing self-Reiki brings me quickly and easily to a state of being much like the centered feeling that comes from walking along the beach at sunrise or sunset. As a mother of four with a full-time teaching schedule, a part-time client schedule, and writing deadlines, I have plenty from which to decompress. After only a few seconds of contact with my body, I begin to feel a warmth like liquid honey flooding through me. The tensions and strains leave my body effortlessly, like silk sliding off my skin. The sensation of the energy flowing from my hands is much more than heat or tingling or vibration. It is similar to the feeling that a child might have when, being cuddled lovingly by his mother, he melts into the delicious comfort of her body. As adults, we need to provide ourselves with comparable comfort and care.

In addition to using the self-Reiki form regularly as a rejuvenating practice, many people choose to put one or both of their Reiki-initiated hands on themselves as they go through their busy days. Talking on the phone, sitting in a meeting, watching

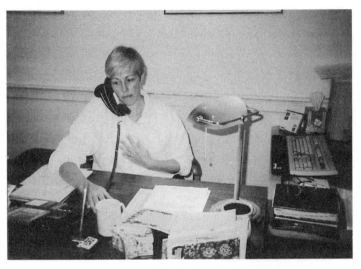

It's easy to include Reiki in daily activities

television, attending a concert, waiting for the traffic light to turn green, standing in the check-out line—these moments or any others are a fine time for doing Reiki. Because the cells bypass the mind in choosing to pull in the universal life energy, Reiki can be received while one's consciousness attends to other issues at hand. An elementary school teacher told us that the school system pays her to do two hours of Reiki on herself every day. "I just keep one hand on my body as I'm walking down the hall, talking to a colleague, helping a student with spelling, or standing on the playground. It's fantastic. I get in my Reiki and it doesn't require any extra time. As a result, I notice that I am more focused during appointments, am able to generate creative ideas and solutions, can more easily access my sense of humor, and have greater stamina overall."

A favorite self-treatment spot for many Reiki practitioners is the heart. When you simply rest the hands on your heart and hold the intention for the highest healing good, transformative vibrations flow into your deepest being, nourishing you and

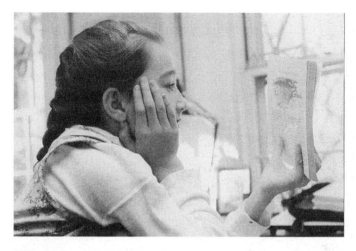

Reiki can be received while one's consciousness attends to other details

assisting you in letting go of all that no longer serves your
unique life purpose. Focusing your mind on compassion and
peace enriches this experience and helps return your heart to its
natural state of lightness and joy. Reiki centers you in your
truth. If you forget the reality of your inner wisdom at any point

Reiki doesn't require any extra time

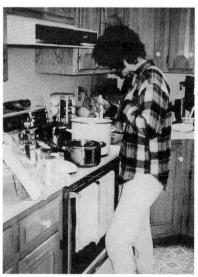

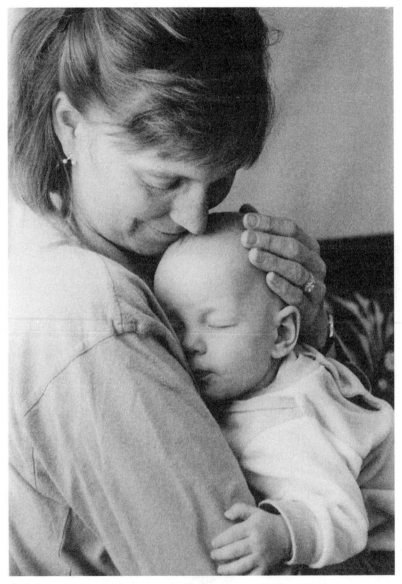

Reiki brings peace and contentment

during the day, putting a hand on your heart instantly reminds you of your connection to the universe and facilitates your living out of this awareness. This profoundly simple and effective tool assists in the healing and transforming necessary for personal evolution. We are each a part of the greater whole of the universe, and each of us comes here with a unique gift and a specific purpose that contributes to the whole. Reiki meets us where we are and gently moves us forward, providing support for doing the work we were born to do. Reiki helps us know our purpose and manifest it with strength, vitality, and ease.

THE REIKI RESOLUTION TECHNIQUE: RESOLVING EMOTIONAL PATTERNS WITH REIKI

At any one moment in time there is a certain and limited reservoir of personal energy from which each of us operates. All physical activities require energy expenditure. Likewise, non-physical efforts such as putting on a brave face when distressed or being nice when feeling miserable also require an output of energy. People who work in the helping professions see what a toll such efforts take on their clients or patients who are in difficult situations and are trying to "keep it all together." An even deeper level of effort is involved in maintaining self-limiting beliefs: habitual ways of viewing life that cause us to feel separate from the whole or not worthy enough to receive what we really long for.

Because patterns—our habitual ways of being—are unconsciously maintained, many people battle against them without really identifying them as antagonists. Some dive deeply into their professional work and become overachievers, ignoring the subtleties of their emotional selves. Others feel a slowly creeping depression take over, usually accompanied by a deepening level of exhaustion. In either case, the energy that is tied up in these limiting patterns of belief and interpretation is not available to us. To the degree that personal energy is involved in maintaining our patterns, the compassion, clarity, and insight that underscore all the efforts of good caregiving are also less available. Our potential is squelched by the power of our limiting patterns. Many healers and others who work in the health-care professions find it important to continually seek their own emotional clarity in order to have a maximal amount of energy available to work with others and to maintain full and satisfying personal lives.

The Reiki Resolution Technique, born out of our work with individuals, groups, and ourselves, is a way to use the mind on a moment-to-moment basis in conjunction with self-Reiki as a means for purposeful soul healing. As we have stated, paraphrasing from the field of new physics, every aspect of reality, including thoughts and emotions, represents energy vibrating at a particular frequency. Being nonmaterial but nonetheless real, all of our feelings and belief systems, unconscious as well as conscious, can be thought of as invisible limbs and, like the limbs of our body, require energy to maintain. Anytime you react to others in a judgmental way—for example, by seeing them as controlling, dependent, demanding, aggressive, or passive—one of your own patterns is simultaneously being revealed to you. For example, a friend whom you consider to be needy and dependent has triggered your own feelings of inadequacy; or a department head whom you feel to be authoritarian has elicited your own tendencies to be controlling and dominating. Those judgments that you project onto others and that rigidify you in your interactions are actually aspects of yourself that are brought into consciousness by the actions and demeanor of the other.

If you do not recognize a pattern as your own, your response is to disown it, to see the personality trait that elicits such judgment as "not mine, but his" (or hers). Actually, your reaction has very little to do with the other person but is more accurately a reflection of an aspect of yourself that needs to be recognized. If you refuse to accept this quality as your own, the lock on your energy is maintained in your efforts to deny it. Similarly, you bind your personal energy by entertaining habitually negative or defeating thoughts such as "I'm not good enough," "There's never enough time," or "I'll never be able to do that." All such thoughts deny you your potential for a satisfying life. When you believe these negative thoughts, seeing them as true and permanent, you disempower yourself.

The energy tied up in maintaining these patterns is unavailable to us in both our personal and our professional lives. A certain amount of exploration of the genesis of these patterns can be useful, but there is a point at which the returns can begin to diminish when we analyze past experiences. Often a residue of the energetic pattern remains in the cells. This residue must be addressed in order for the pattern to be resolved completely. Along with investigating patterns in the light of past events, we can embrace them with self-Reiki, recognizing them as part of us and thereby defusing their power over us.

Recognition is the first step in dissolving a pattern and reclaiming its energy. When you notice yourself being engulfed by your emotions or your thoughts of "I'm not good, smart, accomplished [and so forth] enough," you can take refuge in self-Reiki by putting your Reiki healing hands on your body at the place where you experience the pattern to have its greatest effect on your physical being at that moment. (If you cannot localize the emotion or thought, you can simply place your hands on your heart.) As you give yourself Reiki at this spot, feelings of relaxation and well-being automatically begin to infuse your body as universal life energy streams in. You allow your emotional state to be exactly as it is at that moment instead of trying to deny, justify, or analyze it. With this permission to *be* simply as you are—observing your emotions from a state of witnessing, a state of indifferent awareness—the emotion dissipates. By embracing the pattern, with no requirements that it change or go away, you set the emotion free to follow its own process and transform itself naturally into energy that is more creative and constructive to further your accomplishments and evolution.

When you experience anxiety, for instance, you can dive fully into the illusion that you *are* anxiety and that nothing else exists in your life except this anxiety. You think the anxiety is real. You believe it. When such an energetic pattern is maintained in your mental and emotional bodies for an extended time, you can even create illness, such as colitis or an ulcer, as a result of identifying with it. Reiki acts like a lifeline when you feel yourself drowning in the depths of an intense energetic pattern. As you do self-Reiki, the cells pull in universal life force, flooding the body with a sense of well-being and accessing the body's intrinsic harmony and wholeness. If you focus your mind on this positive sensation, it expands, absorbing your attention. Life is a process of continuous creative flux, and what you attend to with the mind is heightened in your experience.

Sometimes it can be difficult to extricate the mind when it is gripped by a negative mental/emotional pattern. When this happens, you can redirect your mind to think about an uplifting image, such as the soaring flight of a hawk, the beauty of a newborn baby, or the calming rhythm of the ocean's waves. Shifting your awareness away from the negative pattern onto an uplifting thought raises your vibration. Since what you focus on grows and expands, maintaining your awareness on this uplifting image as you do self-Reiki allows you to become more firmly established in the higher vibration. Then, with your hands on your body, you can use the positive feeling generated by your uplifting image to embrace your negative pattern.

If you continue to have difficulty freeing your mind from the conflicted state or emotion, you can facilitate your process by saying the following phrases, in this order, while doing self-Reiki:

1. *"I feel you."* You notice the presence of the emotion.
2. *"I accept you."* You allow the emotion to be simply as it is.
3. *"I embrace you."* You comfort yourself like a mother caring for a hurt child. Saying this phrase with this understanding helps you to recognize that the emotion or thought emerges from a wounded part of you. By saying, "I embrace you," you acknowledge to yourself, "Oh, this is me! Here's another part of me that I can reclaim."

With each step as outlined above, say the phrase with the intention to fully communicate with yourself so that you feel deeply nurtured. Take the time you need to be with and experience fully your emotion or thought. You are listening actively to a very important messenger. Listen with the same attention that you would give to a most significant person in your life. When you begin to dialogue with yourself in this way, you realize how significant an ally you are to yourself in your own healing.

Once you have completed the three steps, let go of them and simply breathe, refocusing your mind on an uplifting image, allowing your awareness to be absorbed into this higher vibration as you continue doing self-Reiki. Do not be tempted to go back and dwell on the negative emotion or thought. Remember—you can choose where you direct your mind.

Living life with awareness of your patterns and implementing the Reiki Resolution Technique is immensely empowering. When you encounter someone or something that sets you off emotionally and thus reveals one of your emotional or psycho-

logical patterns, you have the clarity to recognize the pattern as
part of you, and you have the vehicle to transcend it. No matter
what the pattern is or looks like, you see it without judgment.
You recognize it as part of yourself, honor it by embracing it,
and then return to your uplifted state.

Living in this uplifted state of consciousness is living life from
your center and your truth rather than living inside an illusion, a
reality imposed from the outside. The Reiki Resolution
Technique helps you reconnect with your inner knowing, the
part of you that can acknowledge such a truth as "I am not anxiety. I am whole, powerful, and wise. I am a part of the creative
intelligence of the universe that underlies all life." Because your
cells contain universal life force, they remember the truth of
who they are as they pull in the healing energy. Thus, your
entire being begins to vibrate with this creative power instead of
resonating with the self-limiting pattern.

Because most of us were not raised with the awareness that
we *are* universal life force and that *everything* is energy, including
ourselves, our life choices do not consistently move us toward
wholeness. We can become enmeshed in mental and emotional
patterns that drain our life force and keep us operating on a level
far below our potential as human beings. When we apply the
Reiki Resolution Technique we move from imbalance to
equipoise by using self-Reiki in conjunction with the mind to
get us back in touch with our indwelling power of creation.
When we put our hands on ourselves in a healing way, universal
life energy flows into our body, reminding us of our innate balance and harmony. This is a tangible experience, not a concept
we have to generate with the mind. Reiki gets the momentum
going that allows us to feel better, stronger, and more enlivened,
enabling the mind to shift its focus and elevate our consciousness. As we continue to use the Reiki Resolution Technique to

maintain this state of authentic power, we are gradually freed from our limiting emotions and beliefs and are born into the reality of our true potential.

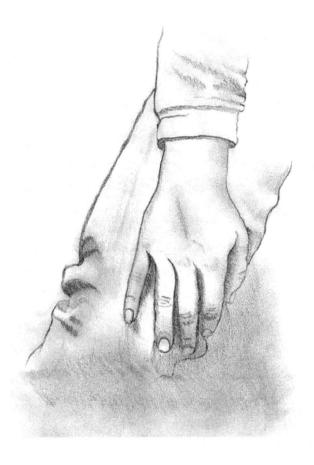

Chapter 4

A
PROGRESSIVE APPROACH
TO WELLNESS

*T*he American health-care system is undergoing dramatic change, challenging institutions to be innovative and to offer the highest quality services while at the same time remaining cost effective. Institutions are turning to complementary therapies as one way to facilitate the demanding tasks of maximizing patient care and minimizing recovery time, while using resources efficiently. Interventions such as Reiki, acupuncture, biofeedback, hypnosis, massage, therapeutic touch, and visualization are gradually becoming integrated into our health-care system. These complementary therapies provide the health-care consumer with broader options and bring a balance and wholeness to standard medical treatment.

Conventional medicine is quite sophisticated in dealing with specific diseases and trauma, but has paid less attention to other aspects of the patient's total wellness, such as how a person feels about his condition. For patients with terminal illnesses, when

51

cure is not part of the care plan, or those with chronic diseases, in which standard medicine has done all it can, integrative medicine—an approach that combines complementary and conventional treatments—is recognized as being helpful for specific physical and emotional problems, as well as contributing to the patient's quality of life.

Therapies that work with the energetics of the mind in relationship to illness are often key to a change in lifestyle, attitude, or point of view.

A primary-care physician referred Martha for Reiki to see whether it would make any difference in her fibroid tumor, since she was fearful of having the necessary surgery. Martha's ability to participate fully in life had been severely curtailed over a two-year period because of the size of the tumor. During the course of the Reiki sessions, Martha's tumor gradually decreased from the size of a softball to a hardball to a golf ball, at which point she decided to learn Reiki to assist her healing between sessions. The gradual reduction of the tumor was accompanied by Martha's increasing recognition of anger regarding her perceived abandonment at a hospital as a child. This insight effected a total reversal of her attitude about surgery. Instead of continuing to fear, Martha began eagerly to arrange the details of her surgery and recovery time, consciously orchestrating a curative experience for herself. Her family rallied around her and showered her with attention. Her surgery went well, turning out to be a celebration and a completion on all levels: physical, mental, and emotional. The Reiki sessions enabled Martha to follow her primary-care physician's initial recommendation.

Holistic therapies not only expand healing possibilities but also are valuable because they are low in cost and require little or no technology to implement. A major concern of most health-care facilities is the bottom line. Adjunct practices such as Reiki are an excellent solution to maintaining high-quality care at minimal cost.

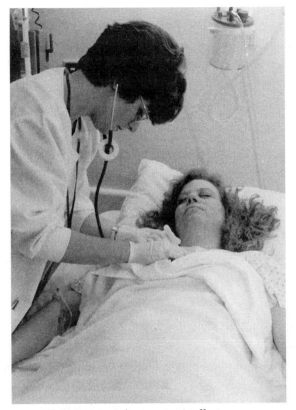

Reiki increases the caregiver's effectiveness

Reiki blends easily with all therapies, because the universal life force is unobtrusive, deeply assistive, and never overwhelming. Since Reiki works beyond the will of the conscious mind, it becomes a part of the health-care professional's full healing capacities, enhancing and expanding her skills without requiring a shift in concentration or attention. Reiki easily joins with and facilitates the client's healing process. An increased flow of life-force energy is available to the patient when touched by a Reiki-trained caregiver. Reiki increases the caregiver's effectiveness and enhances her ability to provide support and exude well-being, thereby augmenting her healing presence.

As Reiki is increasingly recognized by the general public, it is gaining approval and acceptance in mainstream health-care venues. In this chapter we present vignettes highlighting the benefits of Reiki when it is used as an adjunct to standard medical approaches. Reiki has been successfully integrated into clinical settings to complement medical care, hospice care, and psychotherapy.

REIKI IN THE HOSPITAL

Since Reiki requires no specific setting or preparation, it can be utilized in all hospital environments, including outpatient clinics, emergency rooms, intensive-care units, operating rooms, and all other inpatient settings. It can be incorporated into a patient's treatment at any point. Reiki can be used alone or as an adjunct treatment, or it can be integrated seamlessly into the health-care professional's existing medical repertoire. There are many indications for the use of Reiki in hospital settings. It helps relieve stress, agitation, and acute or chronic pain; it is helpful as an aid for sleeping and also as an energizer. It promotes the release of emotions such as grief, anger, or anxiety and provides comfort in palliative care. There are no side effects or contraindications with Reiki; it is noninvasive and appropriate for all segments of the population. Reiki can be performed on a patient while he is lying down, sitting, or standing. The environment can be as quiet as a private room or as stimulating as the emergency room. No adjustment in clothing needs to be made, since Reiki flows through any barrier, including casts.

Because Reiki is not dependent upon the consciousness of the receiver, the patient can be in any mental or emotional state; the patient can even be totally unresponsive, as in a coma. Likewise she can be disoriented, agitated, anxious, or in any other disturbed state and still benefit from Reiki. Either the full Reiki sequence or any part of it can be easily incorporated into

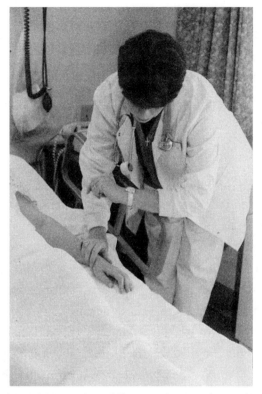

Reiki touch can make a difference when a pulse is taken

the patient's care plan. An extra moment of Reiki touch when the temperature or pulse is taken can make a difference to the patient. When patients are connected to sophisticated monitoring devices that prohibit full access to the body, Reiki can be applied to specific locations with great effectiveness. When Libby and a colleague performed Reiki on hospitalized cancer patients, the high-tech equipment surrounding much of the bed made it impossible to perform the full Reiki treatment. Yet by placing their hands wherever they could reach easily, in just fifteen minutes' time there were noticeable changes in every patient: agitation calmed, eyes gently closed, breathing became deep and regular, and an overall deep relaxation was observed.

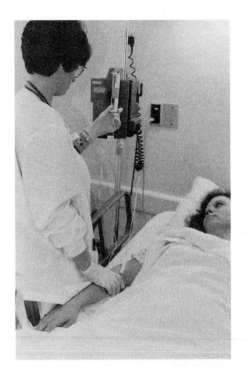

Most nurses we teach use Reiki in routine patient care

A physician who combines Reiki with her practice of surgery told us that patients are less anxious and more calm and relaxed, and they experience less pain and discomfort postoperatively. In most cases, their wounds heal quickly and uneventfully.

Most nurses to whom we teach Reiki use it in routine patient care. Nurses report that certain shifts in patients' conditions are common following Reiki treatment. These shifts include the following:

- Patients "pink up" (i.e., circulation increases).
- Hands and feet warm up.
- Patients sleep calmly and for extended periods.
- Relaxation response is elicited.
- Less time is needed to calm patients following a stressful event.

- Patients have a more positive attitude.
- Patients are more cooperative.
- Patients report decreased pain.

By inducing the relaxation response, Reiki helps in ways that cannot always be quantified but have a visible and very real effect on the patient. For instance, patients undergoing chemotherapy often report less distress and discomfort associated with their treatments when their care plan includes Reiki sessions. Similarly an AIDS patient reported, "Reiki is so gentle. It's the only thing that helps me feel better, rather than adding to my pain." This is not just a matter of *thinking* that there is improvement—the results are real. Patients have increased physical and psychological ability to cope with their illnesses.

> *A teacher was referred for Reiki by a colleague prior to a bone marrow transplant. She had never heard of Reiki, but she was willing to trust her friend that it might help strengthen her for the ordeal ahead. At the completion of the Reiki treatment, which was done in silence, she said that she had experienced a new way of thinking about her cancer. Prior to the Reiki session she had been visualizing the "good" cells killing off the "bad" ones. During the session she experienced a shift in her perspective; she understood the cancer cells to be an integral part of herself that was out of balance and control. She was surprised that she felt love for them. As she accepted these cells, she saw them remembering their purpose and how to function properly. She left the appointment encouraged and feeling better prepared to handle her situation. Five months later, following a successful transplant, she went back to teaching part-time.*

By restoring balance to the energy field, Reiki assists the patient in mobilizing her biological healing resources for recuperation. Reiki can also reduce the need for pharmacologic intervention with respect to both dosage and frequency of administration.

Ann was diagnosed with a detached retina requiring emergency surgery. During the initial exam the ophthalmologist used a probe; it was so painful Ann began sobbing and feeling very frightened. Her partner, Mike, put his hands on her shoulder and gave her Reiki; she gradually relaxed and, much to her amazement, experienced no more pain for the duration of the exam. Following three and one-half hours of surgery, Ann rested comfortably in her room while Mike did Reiki on her bandaged eye. A nurse asked her, "Don't you want something for the pain?" Ann was surprised by the question. Her eye felt gravelly, but there was no pain. The nurse took Mike out into the hall and confided in him incredulously. "Eye surgery is agony," she explained. "It's just unbelievable that she doesn't need pain medication." Ann remained in the hospital for three days; her eye continued to heal quickly and has been fine for the past two years.

Nurses often tell us stories of Reiki's usefulness when standard procedures have been ineffective. They say that patients who haven't gotten relief from anything else often settle down and feel comfortable after they receive a few minutes of Reiki. Their co-workers see that Reiki makes a difference, and often they say, "Go do whatever you do with your hands; it works!" Even though they may not understand Reiki, they are grateful for its presence because it makes everyone's job easier.

Surgeons and nurse anesthetists find Reiki to be helpful pre-, intra-, and postoperatively. The Reiki touch helps the anesthetist to connect quickly with the patient while simultaneously reducing the patient's anxiety regarding the impending procedure. The anesthetist's job is much easier when the patient is less fearful. Because universal life force always works for the highest healing good, and the patient's cells are in charge of the amount received, Reiki never interferes with anesthesia, nor is there any concern about overdose.

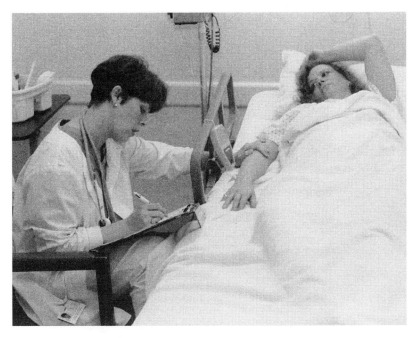

The Reiki touch reduces the patient's anxiety

A fifty-four-year-old woman with a recurrent brain tumor was very anxious during her preoperation preparations, as she was about to undergo disfiguring surgery. In the operating room the nurse anesthetist did Reiki on the patient for several minutes before preoxygenation and again during induction of anesthesia. The patient's vital signs remained stable during intubation and the entire induction process was extremely smooth and easy. The anesthesia staff and the surgeons noticed this; they had expected some difficulty because of the patient's small mouth and history of difficult intubation. Surgery went very smoothly, with little blood loss, and took only five and one-half hours instead of the expected ten to twelve hours. The nurse anesthetist had her Reiki healing hands on the patient's body as often as possible during the operation, and did five more minutes of Reiki at the end of anesthesia. The patient awoke easily and gradually with no coughing or gagging. She was awake, alert, and calm as she was

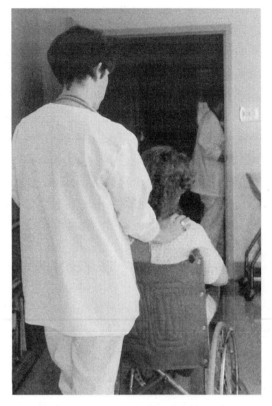

Reiki maximizes everything the nurse does

wheeled to the postanesthesia care unit. The physicians were very pleased and made several comments regarding the short surgical time as well as the uneventful induction process.

Reiki helps the patient regain consciousness in the postanesthesia care unit (the recovery room) following an operation. Reiki maximizes everything the nurse does, enabling her to provide excellent care without taking extra time or distracting her from her extensive responsibilities. A nurse at a Harvard Community Heaith Plan Reiki class commented, "If I had only known Reiki several years ago when my patient came out of anesthesia, saw her partially amputated leg, and burst into tears pleading for me to hold her!"

Upon awakening from anesthesia following a craniotomy for a tumor, a sixty-seven-year-old patient was very agitated and unresponsive to commands. He exhibited extreme movements of his arms and legs; his limbs were somewhat rigid and he waved them about, the motion of his legs being limited only by the safety strap. The nurse on duty placed one hand on his heart to do Reiki; there was an immediate calming effect as his agitation and seizurelike movements ceased, and he became more coherent. After one minute she removed her hand. Five minutes later, his agitation and restless movements resumed. Again she put a hand on his chest with immediate dramatic results—his movements ceased, and he remained calm for the rest of his recovery room stay.

Reiki is particularly useful during the postoperative period to help manage pain and promote healing. Often there is more pain than anticipated and recuperation takes longer than expected. Pain and frustration combined with the fear, spoken or unspoken, that the surgery didn't work, can wear people down. Reiki is a tremendous comfort during the healing process. As one client said with tears of pain and frustration following a shoulder operation, "The doctor doesn't know why I'm still in so much pain, and the physical therapist just keeps saying it's going to take time, but it's already been two months; I just wish the pain would stop." She found that Reiki helped her; even though it did not stop the pain, it made the pain more tolerable.

Ellen was recuperating from a hysterectomy. Following her discharge from the hospital, she developed a bladder infection and was experiencing intense pain. Debilitated by the intensity of the pain, she was unable to urinate and had to use a catheter. Her sister called Maggie and requested Reiki. After a few minutes of Reiki on her head, Ellen began to breathe deeply and drifted off to sleep. Maggie continued to do the head and chest positions of the full Reiki treatment on Ellen for forty minutes. The next day Ellen's husband called Maggie in disbelief.

61

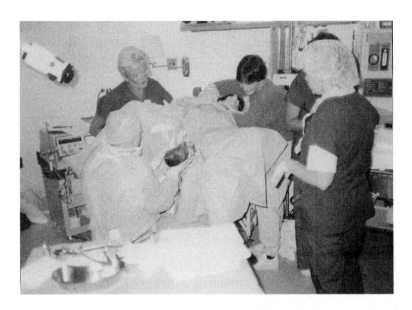

Reiki eases labor and delivery

"What did you do?" he asked. "Not only was Ellen comfortable when she woke up, she was able to urinate normally for the first time in two weeks." Ellen remained free of pain following this one Reiki session, and healed quickly from that point on.

Reiki is also easily incorporated and effective in all practices pertaining to childbirth. Obstetric nurses and midwives find that adding Reiki to their professional skills allows for more holistic clinical practices. Reiki is useful for easing pelvic exams; a few minutes of Reiki on the abdomen or thighs soothes and relaxes the mother-to-be. The use of Reiki during childbirth seems to be associated with reduced use of drugs, shorter labor, and fewer complications. The current medical concept of the birth process focuses mainly on biomechanic factors such as the size and position of the fetus, the mother's pelvic structure, her pattern of contractions, and her medical history. Reiki is one means of bringing the recognition of the human and universal energy fields to the childbirth paradigm. This expansion to a broader theoretical framework allows for the inclusion of Reiki during labor and delivery to help decrease any fear, pain, or discomfort associated with giving birth.

Finally, Pamela Pettinati, M.D., finds Reiki to be extremely beneficial when she performs surgery in Third World countries. On one occasion, when she was preparing for a day of surgery to repair cleft lips and palates and to release burn-scar contractures, a final check of supplies revealed that the oxygen, the medications, the airways, and the monitoring devices were ready to give anesthesia, but the cautery machine had not arrived. When asked what she was going to use to control bleeding, she replied, "Reiki." She did not use the Reiki to cauterize or to stop bleeding; rather, she used Reiki and the bleeding was minimal. She completed long days of operating on babies, young children, and adults. In none of the cases was bleeding a problem, nor did the patients have any other complications.

Dr. Pettinati reports, "The consistent and repeated success of Reiki for these surgical patients defies the odds of bias in patient selection or of merely being lucky. The patients came from remote areas to a central location for surgery. Often they had been seen only once, months earlier, by a local health practitioner, who put that person's name on the list of patients needing surgery. None of them had blood tests preoperatively, since there is no laboratory of any kind. None of the patients had any previous or concurrent knowledge of or exposure to Reiki. In these extreme situations, there is no way to test scientifically the efficacy of Reiki. The stories are necessarily anecdotal, but the sheer numbers and consistency of results are convincing.

"When I was doing surgery in the missions of Latin America, I often became frustrated because we never had enough equipment or supplies. The need was so great, and our ability to

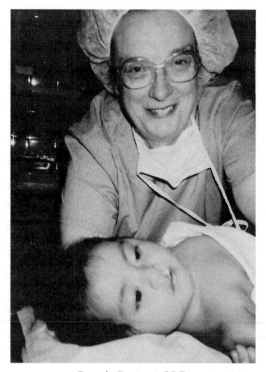

Pamela Pettinati, M.D.

respond seemed so limited. In these situations, Reiki was, indeed, a blessing. Even when I had nothing else to offer to the sick patient and the family, I always had my hands. I could bring consolation, compassion, and the healing touch of Reiki."

Touch is a basic, powerful way to communicate caring. The relaxation response elicited by caring touch underscores the fundamental relationship between touch and health. Reiki provides the caregiver with an expanded awareness of the healing possibilities of each moment of touch. She holds the intention for healing to happen as she goes through her routine assignments, meeting the needs of her patients, knowing that Reiki is available through her hands if her patient chooses to pull it in. The Reiki-trained health-care professional has increased confidence in her ability to cope with whatever situation her patient presents, because she knows the Reiki fuels her touch with universal life force.

As they interact with patients, many professionals find that Reiki improves their interviewing and assessment techniques. A primary-care physician reported an increase in mental clarity and intuition following Reiki class. As he reviews his diagnoses, the ones he refers to as "brilliant" are those in which his intuition operates in tandem with his clinical expertise and knowledge, so this increase in intuitive faculty was a welcomed surprise. He remarked, "In medical school we are trained to approach illness with a cookbook mentality, but that's just not always enough. The only excellent diagnoses are those done from the heart, after all the facts have been weighed. Reiki is a way to put more heart into medicine."

An emergency-room physician with fifteen years of experience took Reiki class on the recommendation of her daughter, who found Reiki to be valuable in her work as a physician's assistant. The physician had no thought of using Reiki in the emergency room and was not looking for any additional skills, but she began to notice some inexplicable changes in her practice of medicine following Reiki class. When she touched patients during her routine medical assessment, their fear and pain often subsided quickly, enabling her to obtain more accurate information in less time. Her questions while she was taking a patient's history were more pertinent, leading directly to the cause of the presenting symptoms. Her increased awareness and heightened intuition helped to support the decisive action so often called for in the emergency room, as when her assessment of a supposed accident revealed child abuse.

This physician has an excellent reputation for accuracy in determining when it is necessary to transport a patient by helicopter to the trauma unit. Because the condition of patients on whom she puts her hands often shifts in ways that she and the emergency-room staff cannot account for, some patients arrive at the trauma unit in better condition than when they left the first hospital. "I'm in danger of crying wolf," she told us, "but better that than that someone not get the attention they need." From a cost containment point of view, she sees the value of Reiki in terms of saving time and reducing work for everyone. Fewer people need to be transported to the trauma unit, and expensive interventions and invasive measures are less frequently called for, because Reiki helps patients stabilize quickly. She contends that her practice of emergency medicine has never been the same since she learned Reiki.

A good number of our Reiki students are nurses who do not have much hands-on time with their patients. Most nurses enter the field of medicine with a deep desire to do healing work, yet they often spend more time working with machines than with patients. The high-tech procedures now carried out in hospitals demand much of the nurse's time, and tension can build up when the workload is so intense that there is not enough time to do all that the nurse would like to do to increase the patient's sense of well-being. This situation can cause immense frustration and contribute to burnout. The Reiki touch is an ideal solution to this dilemma. Reiki enhances the quality of all hands-on interactions, including ones so brief as taking a patient's blood pressure or temperature. These moments of caring Reiki touch, even during routine procedures, increase patients' satisfaction and help to diminish feelings of institutional impersonality. Patients feel as if they are getting more. And they are. This nurturing increases their sense of trust and relationship with the staff, thus making patients more willing to cooperate with their care plan. Reiki satisfies the nurse's innate desire to comfort and

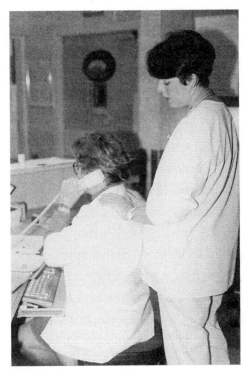

Reiki helps increase cooperation and team spirit among co-workers

nurture, letting the patient know with just a brief touch that someone cares and is trying to help.

Reiki can be used not only to increase patient comfort but also to facilitate communication and well-being among staff. Nurses who practice Reiki with others on their floor or unit report that it helps to harmonize personalities and builds a sense of cooperation and team spirit among coworkers. It is easy to incorporate Reiki into shift changes or floor meetings. While giving their reports on patients at the end of their shifts, nurses often give each other five minutes of Reiki on their shoulders, increasing their focus while releasing the tensions of the day. A floor secretary came to Reiki class because she had experienced a decrease of her chronic arthritis pain as a result of staff members giving her sporadic mini-Reiki treatments on her shoulders and back while she sat at her desk.

Because the Reiki touch nurtures the giver as well as the receiver, as the nurse places her Reiki healing hands on another she receives life force while offering it without having to sacrifice her own well-being. Not only does Reiki increase physical stamina, giving energy to work long hours; it also enables the nurse to maintain mental clarity and emotional stability. Because it supports her on every level, Reiki allows the nurse to do her job in the best possible way. Empowered to integrate caring and nurturing with technological skills, the nurse gets back in touch with her professional passion and purpose. Reiki expands the range of what the nurse can accomplish, increasing job satisfaction and restoring what seems to have been missing from the role of caretaker. Reiki is a way to renew her enthusiasm for her work, helping recreate the original vision that inspired the nurse to choose her profession in the first place.

A nun whose religious ministry is nursing said, "I wish I had my whole career to do over again! Hands-on care is largely delegated to nursing assistants. I regret I cannot do more of it myself. The greatest gift we can bring is our presence. The art of hands-on care can be lost if we do not attend to it, and we must begin with the caretaker. Reiki should be taught to all nursing students." Reiki is a way to bring intentional healing touch back into all aspects of medical treatment.

REIKI IN THE HOSPICE

Reiki can be administered in a variety of hospice settings: a home visit, a hospice room within an institution, or a hospice house. A hospice house is designed to resemble a home, with a bedroom for each resident and a common kitchen and living/dining room. Some hospice houses have guest rooms for relatives.

The Concord Regional VNA-Hospice House, the first hospice

residence in New Hampshire, was designed and custom-built to hospice specifications. During its construction the workers deepened their appreciation for the purpose of their task. They became inspired by the principles of hospice work and the awareness that "their" house would make a difference in the lives of so many people. They often worked overtime and on days off, without pay, to complete the project on time. Community support was abundant, with enthusiastic volunteers and generous contributions from local businesses and individuals. The rooms were decorated with soft, harmonious colors and inviting, comfortable furniture, giving the feeling of a country inn.

Before the hospice house received its first residents, we taught a Reiki class to the staff and volunteers. The purpose was to facilitate bonding and connection as well as to train them so

Reiki offers a stabilizing touch with hospice patients

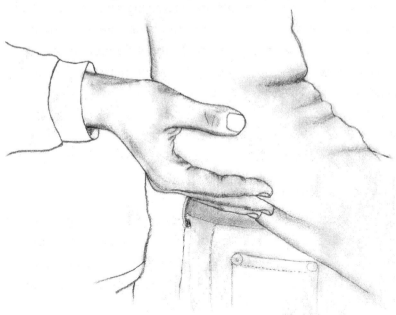

they could provide Reiki for their new residents.

As Reiki-trained hospice staff and volunteers work with clients, Reiki enhances all of their interactions: helping clients to the bathroom, combing their hair, administering medications, reading, feeding, offering a stabilizing touch as they walk down the hall, doing physical therapy, and performing many other daily activities. Reiki transforms these moments of ordinary touch as, in the process of routine activities, the Reiki-initiated touch invites the recipient's cells to pull in more universal life energy. The caretaker does not have to change his behavior when doing Reiki; his actions generally look the same as they did before he learned Reiki. The difference is noticeable, not in the behavior of the hospice worker but in the experience of the client. Because Reiki works beyond the conscious will of either, the helper does not have to think about doing Reiki in order for the client to benefit. One visiting nurse used Reiki with an Alzheimer's patient whose extreme anxiety caused him to clutch at everything. Simple routines took twice as long because she had to detach him repeatedly from the side rails or her arm. She saved herself time, energy, and frustration by giving him a five-minute Reiki treatment before beginning any procedure. He quieted, released his grip, and remained calm. As the nurse said, "Reiki goes beyond being good for people; it really comforts them."

Reiki is particularly useful when the caregiver's standard repertoire does not provide adequate relief from symptoms.

Reiki was included in the care plan for a baby born with neurological damage of an undetermined cause. The physician gave baby Alison a six-month prognosis, warning the young parents not to expect much responsiveness from the child. When the hospice worker began her weekly home visits, she found Alison very agitated and easily disturbed by bright light and noise. The parents reported that she cried for long periods; they were at their wits' end. The hospice worker

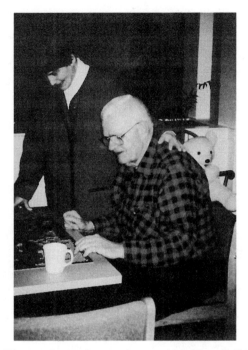

*The practitioner does not have to think about Reiki
in order for the recipient to benefit*

*spent her visits performing Reiki on baby Alison as she held her and
talked with her parents. As the baby pulled in the life-force energy
she became more calm. Over the ensuing weeks the parents noted
with great relief that Alison was less irritable and slept better. During
this time, she also graduated from a feeding tube to a bottle. Currently
Alison is one year old and continues to grow stronger and more alert.
She can follow sounds, identify her parents' voices, and eat soft foods.
Her latest accomplishment is grasping.*

Reiki can look passive, but it is in fact very active as it soothes
pain, nausea, and other physical and emotional conditions.

*A forty-nine-year-old woman with terminal pancreatic cancer looked
forward to the visits from her Reiki-trained home-health aide. As the
aide did Reiki on her shoulder, the patient's eyes closed. She sank
back into the pillow and dropped into a restful state. The patient's*

elderly mother was visibly relieved as Reiki reduced her daughter's pain and agitation.

Reiki not only addresses symptoms but also directly improves quality of life. A dying person's final weeks of life can be fraught with boredom, frustration, loneliness, depression, or fear. Reiki provides comfort and well-being along with deep relaxation and reduction of pain without sacrificing consciousness. Severe pain or fears can be managed more easily and with less medication, leaving the client more alert to deal with the emotional issues of closure with loved ones.

Louise, in the last stages of lung cancer, experienced relief from her pain and her intense fear of dying only when her hospice volunteer did Reiki on her. Libby went to Louise's home to teach Reiki to her and her night nurse so they could do it in the absence of the hospice worker. Her

The Reiki touch provides an avenue for healing and completion

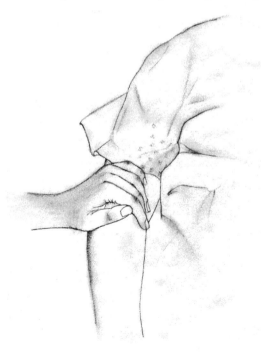

husband, a physician, graciously greeted Libby at the door and stayed long enough to hear an explanation of Reiki. He knew nothing about Reiki and was frankly skeptical, but was willing to invite any treatment that might bring comfort to his wife. With Reiki Louise needed less morphine, enabling her to be more alert during the day and to sleep through the night, providing much needed relief to the entire household.

If the client is unable to articulate his feelings, the Reiki touch provides an avenue for healing and completion.

Reiki proved an invaluable gift for Rebecca to offer her deaf, elderly mother to ease her last three days of life. Her mother had very limited vision, and during the transfer to the hospital her Coke-bottle-thick glasses were lost. Having no hearing and no vision, she seemed to withdraw totally. Wanting to have connection and facilitate her mother's dying process, Rebecca kept her hands on her mother's head,

Reiki is compatible with a hospice's program goals

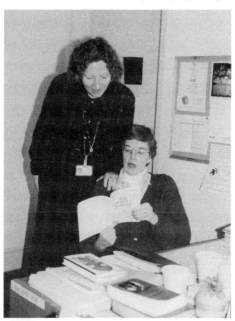

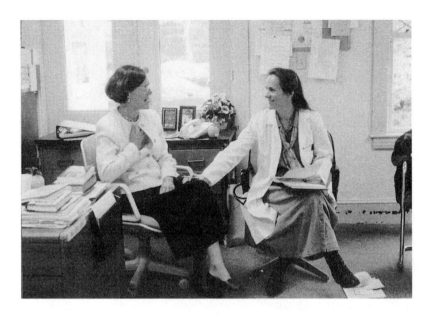

Reiki brings harmony and focus to a hospice staff meeting

shoulder, or heart hour after hour during the three days. Neither Rebecca's legs nor her back, both of which usually bother her when she stands for any length of time, hurt at all. "I consider this truly a miracle because neither my energy nor spirit ebbed during this crisis. I believe this was due to both Reiki and the power of prayer." On the last day, her mother surfaced briefly from her comalike state, looked at Rebecca, emitted a long, engaged sigh, then drew back into herself and passed away.

By supporting the hospice patient through his transition with peacefulness and harmony, Reiki is completely compatible with the hospice's program goals of providing relationship-centered care. The Reiki treatment is gentle, unobtrusive, and always under the client's control. Reiki aligns with the hospice worker's intention that the client feel cared for, secure, and trusting of the caretaker, thereby enabling the client to continue healing and evolving throughout her process of dying. Reiki facilitates the natural flow of this transitional phase of life, giving the caretaker a vehicle for expressing warmth, compassion, and acceptance. As one hospice worker said, "Reiki makes me feel more competent." A rural hospice medical director learned Reiki in order to have something to offer his hospice patients when there was "nothing else to do." It gave him a way to actualize his desire to continue the relationship with the patient, offering excellent care even when the end of life was imminent. "I find myself going to my patients' houses to hold their hands while they die. I've come to learn Reiki so I'll be more effective when I'm holding their hands."

Reiki also helps the hospice worker nurture herself. It is particularly useful in dealing with emotions that can surface as a result of working with dying clients. One hospice caretaker reported, "I do Reiki on myself as I drive to my client's house. It helps me center and focus. During my visit, I often hold my client's hand or shoulder, knowing that she can pull in the energy if she wants to. Afterward, before driving to my next appointment, I just sit in the car for a few minutes doing Reiki on myself to complete the visit."

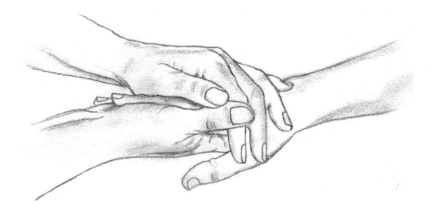

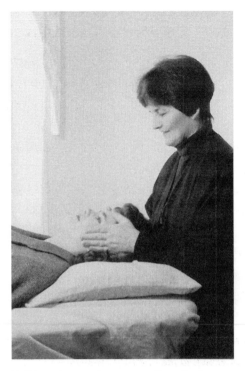

Reiki accelerates the process of psychotherapy

REIKI AND PSYCHOTHERAPY

Many people who seek to resolve their mental or emotional concerns through traditional psychotherapy make considerable progress with verbal process and reach a good understanding of their issues. Yet oftentimes after they achieve a breakthrough insight, an emotional residue remains that still controls their behavior. Reiki accelerates the process of psychotherapy by eliciting additional insights regarding the client's situation as well as by allowing the emotional residue to gently release from the body's cells. The result is a sense of well-being and empowerment.

Caroline, a sixty-two-year-old psychotherapist, had been in therapy herself on and off for many years to deal with her continued feelings of low self-esteem stemming from a history of child abuse. Her peer review was always excellent, and her patients' progress reflected her expertise as a therapist. In spite of this positive feedback, Caroline had continually lived with a judgmental voice inside that said "You're not good enough." Articulate about her issue when she came for Reiki psychotherapy, Caroline said to Libby, "I can't believe that at my age, with my profession and all the work I've done on myself, I'm still plagued by this same old theme!"

The session began in the traditional way with a review of Caroline's history and pertinent facts. Twenty minutes into the session, Libby realized that the direction they were going in was not likely to yield new results. At that point she suggested Reiki. Caroline lay down on the Reiki table and the dialogue continued as Libby moved through the first three Reiki positions on Caroline's head. As Libby's hands were under the back of Caroline's head she asked Caroline where in her body she felt the sense of "not good enough." Caroline's attention was drawn to the intensity of sensation in her abdomen. She then had a sudden flash of imagery suggesting that she had been abused in her grandmother's kitchen when she was three years old; this was an earlier memory of abuse than she had ever recalled before. Caroline described the experience without being overwhelmed, as if she were watching a movie.

Reiki supported Caroline so that she could be in a place of balance from which she could witness her recall without being retraumatized. Of course, all the work she had done previously had prepared Caroline for this breakthrough, which Reiki facilitated by helping her access the preverbal information stored below conscious memory. Libby and Caroline met for a few more sessions to process Caroline's experience and bring it to resolution. In a short time the familiar feeling of low self-esteem completely disappeared.

The inclusion of touch in the psychotherapeutic setting is

something each therapist must assess for himself, given his client's condition, history, and perceived level of trust. While touch is often contraindicated for sexually abused clients, there are case histories demonstrating the effectiveness of Reiki in helping these clients access and gently release stored memories, facilitating and accelerating the course of therapy. This can often be done without the client's having to relive the original trauma. The safe, compassionate nature of Reiki provides for a curative experience of touch, in contrast to the kind of touch associated with the trauma.

During Reiki class, Angie was captivated by the healing quality of the touch she received. She left class eager to do self-Reiki—hungry for what Reiki had to offer—although she couldn't articulate exactly why she so deeply wanted this experience.

In a bookstore several days later, Angie was surprised to find herself reading a book on child abuse. Stunned, she realized the story was her own. She bought The Courage to Heal *and began working through it page by page. As she delved more deeply into the material she realized she needed support and went in search of a Reiki psychotherapist.*

During the next several months, self-Reiki was a constant support for Angie between her weekly Reiki psychotherapy sessions with Libby. By the end of seven months, she was able to perceive her mother's actions with understanding and forgiveness—something she had thought she would never be able to do. After ten months, the energy that had been caught up in coping and surviving was now available to Angie for creative expression. Much to her surprise and delight, she began drawing portraits.

A year later, her weekly session became bimonthly and therapy ended after fourteen months. "My friends were amazed to see the timid, hesitant, shy introvert be replaced by a more relaxed, confident, authentic me. The personality traits I thought I was stuck with turned out to be old ways of thinking and being that I had once needed for survival but was now able to shed."

Experience indicates that a broad spectrum of clients in psychotherapy can benefit from Reiki. The decision to include Reiki in the treatment plan cannot be determined solely on the basis of diagnosis. Equally important are the relationship of the therapist and client, the client's perception of Reiki, and the timing of the introduction of Reiki. Additionally, state law and professional association guidelines need to be consulted before including Reiki in the psychotherapeutic context. Many psychotherapists who want to include a body component in their practice become licensed as ministers, since most states allow clergy to touch clients in the process of their healing ministry. While the issue of touch in the psychotherapeutic process is controversial these days, it is nevertheless obvious that the inclusion of Reiki, when appropriate, can encourage full resolution of difficult patterns.

Based on my (Libby's) training at the Simmons College School of Social Work and my experience as a medical social worker at Massachusetts General Hospital, the fundamental principle guiding my Reiki psychotherapy practice is that all healing comes from within. The client is not fragile. Indeed, he or she is powerful and whole, having all the answers within. Reiki supports the accessing of this inner wisdom.

I welcome each client with love and respect, and create a trusting relationship by working from these principles:

- Come from my heart, not my head
- Relate to the essence of the client, not the personality
- Listen without judgment
- Be willing not to know
- Let go of attachment to results

This safe, sacred connection becomes the context within which all possibilities for healing and transformation can arise.

Within this context I offer up our work together for the highest healing good, trusting in the wisdom of the body, mind, and emotions of both my client and myself.

Client appointments last an hour to an hour and a half. We spend part of the session talking, and the client spends the rest of the time on the Reiki table. Once on the Reiki table, the client is covered with a light flannel sheet, as if to say "It's okay to nestle under the covers and do your healing work. You're safe. You can trust your process." The Reiki part of the session can include dialogue or can be conducted in silence, allowing the client to integrate what has been focused on and to access additional insights. As the session progresses, the client usually becomes deeply relaxed and sometimes even falls asleep.

This time on the table is not only an opportunity for the client to pull in the universal energy but also an invitation to release any residual traumas. These residues usually release easily and gently, without inducing the client into processing the issue one more time. This release is never overwhelming because at a deeply unconscious level the client is in charge of how much and how fast he pulls in the energy. The therapist does not regulate or control the flow of Reiki to the client.

Since it is the client who does the actual healing work, the therapist's role is that of facilitator. The therapist acts as a midwife for the client's healing process, which necessitates *being* more than *doing*. Yet relinquishing the role of doer does not mean that the therapist abdicates responsibility in the situation. The therapist's presence is essential: in addition to being a vehicle through which the universal life energy enters, the therapist stands guard over the client's process, holding the intention that healing happen for the client's highest good and guiding the process with questions and comments based on traditional psychotherapeutic principles.

Reiki psychotherapy is definitely a collaborative effort involving the universal life force, the client's inner healing resources, and the therapist's skillfulness and intention. Unconditional love is the essence of this simple, powerful healing method, the purpose of which is to bring balance, harmony, and wholeness to all aspects of the being.

We have taught Reiki to numerous psychotherapists whose goal in combining Reiki with their therapy practice is to enrich and facilitate their sessions with clients. Susan Golden, a psychologist and Reiki student of ours, interviewed psychotherapists about how Reiki was benefiting their clients. All the therapists Susan interviewed are highly experienced, with ten to thirty years in the field and well-established, successful practices. Their combined client base is diverse and includes many survivors of extreme trauma. Some keep Reiki tables set up in their offices; others use pillows or chairs for Reiki treatments. Selected comments from these interviews will help to highlight Reiki's effectiveness as a tool for therapeutic support.

One therapist describes her experience with an incest survivor with whom she has worked for over three years. "He would often get into the pain and the memories and dwell there. With Reiki he started to move through his pain. In using Reiki I find clients really do move through their issues and problems. They make important connections on the mental, spiritual, emotional, and physical levels and have more uplifting outcomes overall. They often move in one session from a level of pain to a place of resolution. I'm amazed by the speed of their progress, and I'm working much less hard." Another therapist comments, "Reiki really helps with those clients who are disassociated from the body and are living in the head. It cuts to deeper emotions. They reach a different level, understanding things more intuitively and breaking patterns of abusive and

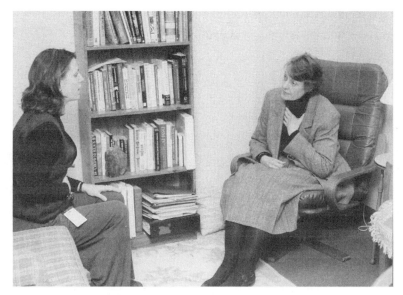

Reiki brings increased clarity to supervision

unfulfilling relationships." Another therapist describes a woman's trauma of separation from her mother, when she was two years old, that impaired her ability to experience intimacy in significant relationships. When she got close to her feelings of loss and abandonment her breathing would become shallow. Anxious, she would find it hard to stay with her feelings. The therapist comments, "Doing Reiki on her allowed her to stay with her feelings longer, to meet them instead of dancing away from them."

Reiki increases clients' capacities to generate imagery, to see and tell their stories, to recognize how their stories are currently expressed in their lives, and to change the expected outcome. As one of the therapists reports, "I put my hands on my client's knee. As I did Reiki I asked her to close her eyes and tell me what she experienced. She saw an image that was the key to an important personal story, a metaphor for her experience. She was able to transform the image and change the story in a way that created room for change in her life." Another therapist describes her work with a client who had a large number of physical problems, including a pain that felt like a hole in her gut. The therapist did Reiki on the client's abdomen at the spot she indicated. As the client's cells pulled in the universal life force, she recalled the experience of a previous injury: her current medical problems seemed to be related to the energetics of this physical problem that had occurred in the past. In a few weeks her symptoms were completely gone. She felt Reiki was a boost to her healing.

Summarizing her interviews, Dr. Golden noted three key results in integrating Reiki and psychotherapy:

1. The therapists reported a deepening of the therapeutic work and a quicker reestablishment of emotional equilibrium. Clients were less likely to be overwhelmed by painful material and were more able to stay with their feelings and achieve resolution.

2. Clients' imagery became more accessible and clear. They experienced an increased ability to recover memory.

3. Clients were better able to make connections on the emotional and physical levels that were productive in their therapy. Reiki was particularly useful in exploring both the meaning and the secondary function of somatic symptoms.

In conclusion, there were differences in how and when the therapists in this study used Reiki in their sessions. Nevertheless, all of the practitioners interviewed clearly feel that Reiki is a useful and positive addition to their practice of psychotherapy, greatly enhancing its effectiveness. They report that using Reiki with their clients is energizing rather than draining and significantly reduces the level of stress they experience as therapists.

Many report becoming more spontaneous and trusting of their intuition, and some feel that using Reiki helps them develop more detached compassion. Using Reiki in a psychotherapeutic setting benefits both client and practitioner, opening both to the flow of universal life energy. As one therapist summarizes it: "Reiki is healing, calming, and restoring for me as well as my clients."

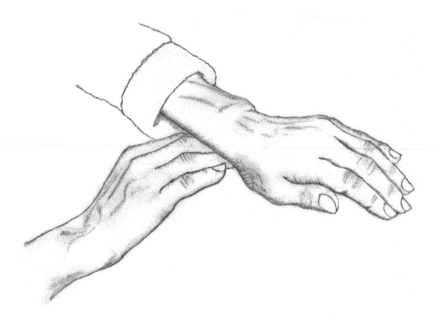

Chapter 5

VISIONS FOR THE FUTURE: REIKI AND THE PARTNERSHIP MODEL OF CARE

*C*omplex procedures, surgery, and sophisticated drugs—invaluable when needed—do not provide a cure for every medical problem and are too expensive to dispense casually. We are on the brink of a new era in medicine, living a moment in history that invites us to expand our collective consciousness to allow for a much wider understanding of the forces of life and how these forces shape and invigorate the human body. At this moment in our cultural history, we can choose to hold fast to our existing paradigm of health and disease: one that encourages the use and development of technology and sophisticated procedures, one that makes the art of medicine a business increasingly able to fully service only the elite in our society. Or we can choose to begin fashioning a health-care system that provides services that are simple and inexpensive when they can be and complex and expensive only when they must be.

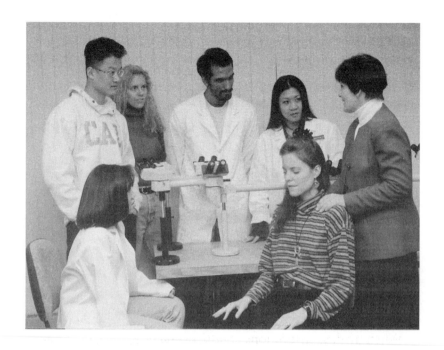

Teaching Tufts medical students

To this end, we are teaching Reiki to health-care professionals in a variety of settings, and their feedback is exceedingly positive. Although the majority of our students working in standard
medicine are nurses, an increasingly greater number of physicians are learning Reiki. Often the physician notices that certain
nurses have an outstanding ability to reach patients, producing
more effective healing in a shorter time. Upon investigation,
they discover that these nurses are Reiki-trained and, being curious, they enroll in a Reiki class themselves to see firsthand what
benefits it might offer. Some now write orders for Reiki.

Endorsement of Reiki by the physician opens the door for
more people to experience its benefits. For example, after
one physician, Patrick Cleary, attended a meeting of hospice
medical directors where we presented an introduction to Reiki,
he requested that a class be organized for hospice staff,

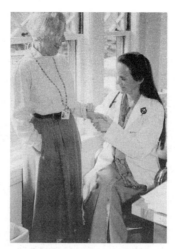

Endorsement of Reiki by the physician opens the door
for more people to experience its benefits

volunteers, and oncology nurses at the hospice he directs.

When medical institutions conduct surveys to measure how well they are meeting patients' needs, some of the key areas addressed include satisfaction regarding the health-care provider's attention, concern, and availability, as well as the range and cost of services. In response to economic realities and consumer demand, and in order to serve diverse populations, medical institutions are being challenged to keep step with the progress being made in medical research while at the same time providing the widest range of quality health-care options at an affordable cost. Our current health-care crisis requires the development and structuring of an expanded, multidimensional therapeutic system that combines the best elements of both conventional and complementary medicine—one that blends art, caring, and ancient wisdom with technical and scientific expertise. This integrated network would offer a wider range of excellent treatment options for all conditions and a correspondingly wider range of costs. Such a diverse system, synergistically strengthened by each modality, would expand the present authoritarian

medical model into a readily accessible, more comprehensive
and participatory health-care system to assist the patients' healing process. United by the common goal of best possible patient
care, these disciplines would be encouraged to rise above individual differences in order to coalesce into a partnership that
embraces a philosophy of treating and caring for the whole
being.

When discussing the possibility of blending complementary
therapies with conventional medicine, allopathic health-care
providers often point to the lack of valid scientific research to
prove the efficacy of these therapies. Well-designed studies to
determine the benefits of complementary therapies are an
essential prerequisite to endorsement for alternative modalities
from the medical community. Still, as a biological researcher
from Massachusetts General Hospital said to us, "The issue,
however, is not how or why they work but *that* they work." His
comment seems to be substantiated by the $10.3 billion that in
1990 was paid out-of-pocket to providers of unconventional
therapies. In the same study it was reported that seventy-two
percent of the people who used alternative therapies did not
report these visits to their doctors.[1] Withholding this information creates added stress for the patient; open communication
between patient and physician is essential in the determination
of which therapies would be appropriate to include in the
course of a person's treatment. Dialogue between patients and
their physicians ensures more comprehensive care and widens
the field of awareness of the role of nonconventional therapies
in the healing process. As physicians hear firsthand testimonies
from their patients concerning the benefits of Reiki, they are
often more willing to investigate Reiki because they know that
anything that can help to control symptoms has a place in a
patient's overall care plan.

In October 1995, the Office of Alternative Medicine and the Office of Medical Applications of Research, National Institutes of Health, convened a Technology Assessment Conference on Integration of Behavioral and Relaxation Approaches into the Treatment of Chronic Pain and Insomnia. The conference concluded, "A number of well-defined behavioral and relaxation interventions are now available, some of which are commonly used to treat chronic pain and insomnia. Available data support the effectiveness of these interventions in relieving chronic pain and in achieving some reduction in insomnia. . . . Although the literature demonstrates treatment effectiveness, the state of the art of the methodologies in this field indicates a need for thoughtful interpretation of the findings as well as an urgency to translate them into programs of health care delivery.

"Although specific structural, bureaucratic, financial, and attitudinal barriers exist to the integration of these techniques, all are potentially surmountable with education and additional research, as patients shift from being passive participants in their treatment to becoming responsible, active partners in their rehabilitation."[2]

As we await additional research results, what else can be done to promote the understanding and acceptance of complementary forms of healing? In addition to research, education must also be promoted. Often after learning Reiki and experiencing its effectiveness, professionals want their colleagues to know about it. A director of social services at a large visiting nurse association was so enthusiastic following class that she presented a Reiki introductory program to thirty nurses, most of whom were veterans with more than twenty years' experience. Their evaluations were extremely high. The director repeated the presentation for the home health aide department, and nineteen attended. Their positive response sent a strong message to the nurse education coordinator. As a result, we taught Reiki to the ten members of the social service department as well as several nurses and physical therapists.

Groups of health-care professionals such as the Mind-Body Medicine Group at Massachusetts General Hospital are gathering within institutions in order to educate themselves about holistic healing modalities. The Englewood (New Jersey) Hospital and Medical Center presents a bimonthly lecture series on holistic and complementary healing modalities which is attended by nurses and other medical professionals from Englewood and adjacent health-care institutions. Not only are these groups educating themselves; some are also spearheading the dialogue regarding research initiatives.

Until recently, alternative therapies have not been included in medical school curricula in the United States, and few physicians have had extensive personal experience with them. (In Europe, where complementary therapies are more often incorporated into the medical process, many medical schools include courses in these interventions.) Progressive medical schools in the United States are now beginning to include education in complementary therapies in their curricula. The first textbook on alternative medicine, "Fundamentals of Complementary and Alternative Medicine," is being used at the University of Virginia School of Medicine at Charlottesville, and is under review at several other schools. Several medical educators are emerging as pioneers in the field of medical education. Andrew Weil, M.D., Assistant Professor of Clinical Medicine at the University of Arizona School of Medicine, is in the process of establishing the Center for Integrative Medicine, a postgraduate fellowship program described as combining "the best ideas and practices from all available systems of treatment into cost-effective therapies that aim to stimulate the natural healing potentials of the human organism."[3] In Dr. Weil's words, "As standard medicine reaches the limits of its economic viability, it is in everyone's interest to sort out the best ideas and practices of alternative medicine and work to integrate them into a new model of health care."[4]

Dartmouth Medical School offers "Evaluating Complementary Medicine," an eight week elective taught by three faculty members: Dale Gephart, M.D., Bob Rufsvold, M.D., and Seddon Savage, M.D. At Georgetown University School of Medicine, James Gordon, M.D., professor of psychiatry and head of the advisory council to the Office of Alternative Medicine at the National Institutes of Health, teaches a class in "Healing Partnerships," providing students with an overview of alternative options. At Tufts University School of Medicine, Glenn Rothfeld, M.D., teaches a similar class called "Complementary Healing Systems," and the student-run Humanistic and Holistic Health Care organization at Tufts University School of Medicine invited us to present an introduction to Reiki to first- and second-year medical students. Following the introduction several of the medical students asked to learn Reiki and organized a class. Because of the students' enthusiasm for Reiki, the administration invited us to return to teach Reiki as a pre-clinical selective. One second-year student commented, "If we have an explanation and experience of complementary therapies like Reiki during our first and second years of medical school we will be more likely to include them in our practice." Harvard Medical School's Department of Continuing Education and the Mind/Body Medical Institute, Deaconess Hospital, sponsored "Spirituality and Healing," a course in which discussions of physical pain were emphasized because "it is incompletely treated by current medical practices." Harvard Medical School's Continuing Education Department also offered "Alternative Medicine: Implications for Clinical Practice," under the direction of David Eisenberg, M.D.

When the College of Physicians and Surgeons at Columbia University accepted a grant to establish the Richard and Hinda Rosenthal Center for Alternative/Complementary Medicine at the university, Dr. Herbert Pardes, dean of the faculty of medicine, said, "A university teaching hospital is exactly the place you can look at things that may be offbeat. We should bring a rational approach to these therapies. The public will be served."[5] These educational institutions are to be acknowledged for their dedication to excellence. By expanding medical education, these schools are laying the foundation for enhancing the practice of medicine.

Another groundbreaking physician, a man cited by the *New York Times* as the most accomplished cardiothoracic surgeon in the country, is Mehmet Oz, M.D., who invites hands-on healers into the operating room at Columbia-Presbyterian Medical Center to work with the patient and participate as part of the operating-room team as he performs surgery.[6] Impeccably skilled in Western medical science, Dr. Oz recognizes the limitations of the allopathic model and is exploring the contribution of energy healing to the physical, emotional, and psychological condition of his patients. Dr. Oz's strong sense of ethics and his commitment to providing the best possible patient care outweigh any concerns about criticism. He has stepped outside the impediment of professional bias in order to participate fully in a scientific endeavor to observe objectively the facts of this marriage between conventional and complementary approaches to healing.

Responding to the growing interest in complementary therapies to supplement conventional medical interventions, some cutting-edge hospitals are beginning to include in their community education programs courses in tai chi, yoga, Reiki, meditation, and relaxation techniques. The goal of these self-reliance health-care programs is to help people stay healthy by means of self-care modalities that encourage connecting with the life-force energy, so they can increase their physical well-being and lessen the chances of needing expensive medical services in an emergency situation that could have been averted by personal actions toward wellness. Wellness programs are a cost-effective strategy for health maintenance. In looking for ways to achieve and sustain a state of wellness, both the medical establishment and health-care consumers can look to the power and the simplicity of Reiki.

Our cultural mind is making a gradual but profound shift toward considering the responsibility for healing as belonging to the patient himself. Progressive educational and group-support programs are being established to inform participants about complementary as well as conventional therapies so that people can utilize the best of both approaches. An example of such an undertaking is the Wellspring Cancer Help Program in New Hampshire. This educational and group-support effort is modeled after the Commonweal Cancer Help Program in Bolinas, California, which is endorsed by oncologists, psychotherapists, and other health professionals and was featured in the PBS documentary "Healing and the Mind." Wellspring seeks to "support and encourage each individual's capacity to heal through a program that consciously reduces stress while activating the individual's connection to their source of inner wisdom and healing."[7] Wellspring accomplishes its purpose by offering a variety of experiences in complementary therapies, including mind/body meditation and progressive relaxation exercises, imagery, yoga, massage, and various forms of therapeutic touch. Participants can also engage in self-exploration sessions, using art, music, poetry, dreams, and a sand tray. Regular attendance to self-care practices or self-initiated healing routines reflects a recognition of the indwelling energy that moves each person toward wholeness.

Bob Rufsvold, M.D., the president and medical director of Wellspring Foundation of New England, offers Reiki sessions to each of the participants of the week-long residential retreat. He finds Reiki very effective in deepening relaxation and diminishing pain. After experiencing the beneficial effects of Reiki, several graduates of the Wellspring program have requested additional sessions or have taken classes to learn how to do Reiki on themselves.

In the past few years several health insurers have recognized that nonconventional treatment options can save them money; for example, several sessions of chiropractic or acupuncture cost much less than surgical intervention. Some insurers are even creating alternative-care benefit packages for consumers. Mutual of Omaha found Dr. Dean Ornish's lifestyle-based healthy-heart program to be an effective money-saving alternative to more invasive treatment. As a result, fifteen other insurance companies are now supporting Ornish's program as a viable alternative to bypass surgery.

Even though Reiki is still not covered routinely by most insurance companies, in 1991 Libby was approached by Blue Cross/Blue Shield of New Hampshire with a proposal to provide coverage for Reiki sessions for a twenty-three-year-old diabetic patient with multiple hospital emergency admissions. This proposal was the outcome of a case conference requested by the insurance company because of its concern about the high costs resulting from the patient's numerous medical crises. The conference was attended by many of the medical personnel involved in the patient's care, including the psychiatrist, social worker, primary-care physician, and nurse practitioner. All were seeking a solution to the negative impact of these crises on the patient's physical condition as well as on her emotional attitude. In presenting the patient's history it was noted that Reiki helped stabilize her blood sugar levels, soothe her neuropathy, and manage the emotional aspects of her diabetes, and that she had fewer crises when she maintained regular Reiki appointments. The insurance company's decision to cover the Reiki sessions turned out to be a wise one. Reiki continued to help stabilize the patient's condition, reducing the number of hospital emergency admissions and thereby saving money for the insurance company.

Vision: Reiki and the Caregiving Team

The hospital environment is an excellent arena in which to experience the results of integrating complementary therapies with standard medical practices. In a hospital where the staff, the patients, and the patient's loved ones were Reiki-trained, the quality of patient stay would be enhanced and the length of stay likely shortened. Clinicians using Reiki would be better able to keep up with the fast pace and demands of their jobs. Reiki-trained family members would be able to take a more active part in the patient's care and treatment, reducing demands on the primary caregiver. A patient who can practice self-Reiki feels more in control of his situation and less dependent on his caregiver. Reiki often reduces the need for pain medication, resulting in fewer side effects and a feeling of empowerment on the part of the patient from having participated in his own recovery. Reiki facilitates not only the hospital course of treatment but also the period of convalescence at home.

Establishing twenty-four-hour "Reiki rooms" where patients could receive Reiki would be a concrete step toward fulfilling any health-care institution's commitment to providing more sensitive patient care, and would signal its willingness to take into account the full spectrum of a patient's needs. Unfamiliar hospital routines, new faces, intimidating and often painful procedures, worry, and fear can aggravate the stress of any condition. Going to the Reiki room for a session would allow patients to relax and feel comforted, encouraging more positive attitudes. Setting up and organizing these Reiki rooms would create little additional cost for the hospital. The Reiki rooms could be staffed by volunteers, a resource that hospitals currently use in nearly every department. Volunteers not only provide support at a great financial savings to the hospital but also add an ambiance that comes with recognizing the innate human desire to care for another. Patients would know that the Reiki-trained volunteers were there because they wanted to help the patients feel cared for and comfortable.

Likewise, health-care providers could also benefit from time in the Reiki room. Ten minutes of Reiki could help a hospital professional with many responsibilities feel less overwhelmed and become more centered, and thus be more available to patients and colleagues. If hospital staff availed themselves of the Reiki room on a regular basis, it would make a dramatic difference in their energy levels, creativity, and coping abilities, helping transform the hospital into a place of true healing for all. Stressed colleagues might remind each other to visit the Reiki room for self-renewal and relaxation.

Lengthy hospital procedures with costly overnight stays are being replaced when possible by hospital-based outpatient surgical procedures. Whether following same-day surgery or discharge after a period of stay in the hospital, knowing how to do self-Reiki as well as how to take medication would benefit any patient's healing process. Reiki provides the patient with a powerful tool to extend and enhance the healing intention of a surgical procedure. With Reiki the patient actively shares in the responsibility for the success of the procedure rather than passively expecting the surgeon to "fix" him. Practicing Reiki on the suggestion of the physician would reinforce a patient's sense of his own responsibility for healing and his sense of partnership with the medical team.

VISION: REIKI AND COMMUNITY OUTREACH

By the year 2030 it is estimated that in America the percentage of people over age sixty-five will exceed the percentage of people under age eighteen. Social interaction and participation in community activities are important factors in counteracting the negative effects of the aging process. The sense of feeling needed and making a contribution is critical in maintaining self-esteem and promoting quality of life. Reiki clinics provide a structured context in which participants receive universal life force for healing on all levels. One small town has a Reiki clinic in its recreation center where Reiki practitioners have gathered for three years to offer Reiki treatments to each other and to the community. Because the group that started this particular Reiki clinic is mainly composed of hospice volunteers, they frequently invite the family members of their hospice clients to receive a Reiki treatment, helping to revitalize and strengthen them as they handle the death of their loved one.

Following the community-service model of Reiki clinics currently in existence, Reiki clinics staffed by senior citizens would serve the needs of the community while giving older adults a meaningful way to contribute to society. These clinics could be located in any number of places, including rehabilitation facilities, hospice houses, and senior citizen centers. Providing an antidote to the rampant isolation and loneliness in our touch-starved culture, these clinics could become focal points in the community—places of refuge for relationship and caring. They could provide participants with a heightened sense of well-being and an increased capacity to function in daily living. Following the Reiki protocol, the staff of elders would be making a difference while simultaneously meeting a basic need to connect with others.

VISION: REIKI AND THE LIFE/DEATH/LIFE CONTINUUM

Perhaps in no other aspect of life has our current medical paradigm had a more devastatingly antiholistic effect than on our approach to death. Once viewed as a natural, deeply significant part of life, the process of death has been stripped of its beauty and power and reduced to a medical failure, robbing the dying individual of the sacredness of her passage.

As with hospitals, Reiki can and should be taught to hospice staff, patients, and their loved ones to facilitate this natural and inevitable phase of life. Self-Reiki is a powerful means by which the patient can express her autonomy and fully participate in her passage from this life. Reiki helps the hospice patient to manage pain and to deal with any fears and anxieties about dying. Self-Reiki can be used by the patient to reduce her pain medication, enabling her to be more alert and thus able to connect and complete processes with others. Many of the limitations associated with this stage of life, such as physical weakness, lack of concentration, or depression do not impede one's ability to do Reiki, since Reiki only requires that the patient lay her hands anywhere on her body. With Reiki the hospice patient is empowered to meet her own needs, especially when others are not available—often the case at night or during quiet moments. At these times sadness or fear can intensify. When that happens the dying person can put her hands on herself and relax inside the extraordinary comfort of Reiki.

Reiki is equally supportive for family members and friends as their loved one is dying. The sense of helplessness that can be present in terminal situations is made more tolerable for the extended family because they realize they have something of value to offer when there is nothing else that can be done. Instead of anxiously wringing their hands, they can do Reiki on their loved one as well as on themselves. Reiki gives them a reason to touch, transmuting sadness into loving action. As the universal life force flows, it calms and soothes the providers as well as the patient. Anxieties decrease, enabling both the patient and those close to him to focus more on accepting and understanding the impending death, thus facilitating the dual processes of grieving and letting go. When this final phase spans many weeks, the stress on family members and friends can be enormous. Doing Reiki on each other provides invaluable nurturing and support.

As those in the baby-boomer generation mature, they are demanding greater consciousness around the processes of aging and dying. The impending shift in our country's demographics may create a cultural shift in which the valuable opportunities presented by death are fully explored and acknowledged. With the recognition that death has the potential to be one of the most healing and transformational events of life will come the desire to take advantage of this opportunity. Dr. Elisabeth Kubler-Ross and Ondrea and Stephen Levine, prominent spokespersons for the healing potential in the process of dying, emphasize that this final stage of life offers profound opportunities for growth. Yet, because our society has not become adept at dealing with this event, we need tools for support. Reiki is one such tool. Loved ones who choose to participate more actively in the patient's dying process may feel awkward or inadequate, especially in trying to find words to express their feelings. The healing power of Reiki caring touch eliminates the burden of having to articulate emotions. Touching and giving Reiki communicates the depth of caring and connection without the need to use words.

As our culture embraces the wholeness of life, people will experience more freedom in how they honor and even celebrate life's final healing opportunity. The dying and those who love them will have alternative and humane options to aggressive medical procedures—last-ditch attempts at prolonging life that are often invasive and come at an exorbitant cost, but have little promise of cure or even improvement in quality of life. These medical interventions, born of the pernicious trend to *do* something, sometimes cause negative side effects that further compromise the patient's quality of life, producing a result that is the exact opposite of what was intended by physician and family. Often these interventions drain the patient's life force, making that energy unavailable for closure and expanding consciousness—the designated tasks of this final stage. As Jack McCue, M.D., writes, "Viewing dying as an independent diagnosis in patients who are obviously undergoing terminal declines from aging and chronic diseases can facilitate communication about spiritual and palliative care needs, which tend to be neglected in the medicalized view of dying."[8] When we allow dying to be a diagnosis, we create the possibility that Reiki and other complementary therapies will be acceptable and viable options to more invasive procedures. This provides the patient and family with a continuum of choices to support them as they meet death with awareness and courage. The dying deserve to be heard, acknowledged, and touched as they move through this passage with consciousness and dignity.

VISION: REIKI AND HUMAN EVOLUTION

Though Reiki is not easily explained, it is easily experienced, and the experience opens us to new possibilities for achieving optimal well-being. We are advocating combining the best of conventional medicine with the best of complementary modalities to yield a superior health-care system that addresses not only the absence of symptoms and disease but also the development of good health based on total care for the whole person. The wisdom and effectiveness of this approach are illustrated by the story of Nathan, a three-year-old boy diagnosed with a very rare rhabdoid tumor of the kidney. Eight and one-half hours of surgery were required to remove the kidney and tumor. After undergoing a year of chemotherapy and other conventional as well as complementary therapies, including Reiki, his doctors report that Nathan has had the only recovery they have seen out of all twenty-nine such cases in the country since 1988. His only side effect was hair loss; he suffered no mouth sores, hearing loss, eye troubles, or digestive problems. Nathan's latest MRI scan showed that he was completely free of cancer, with no inflammation of his lymph nodes. He is now four years old, has learned Reiki, and is happily attending preschool. Reiki was a part of all that was used in Nathan's care plan; everything together contributed to Nathan's recovery.

Energy medicine is an idea whose time has come. More information on how it works will be available as research progresses; meanwhile, its effectiveness is not dependent on our understanding of it. Incorporating Reiki with conventional health care not only assists with curing the curable, but also provides a solution for caring for the incurable. Because Reiki facilitates the body's creative ability to heal itself, dramatic healing shifts can occur when Reiki is included in one's daily self-care routine or is part of a medical treatment plan. Although we have discussed Reiki using its formal definition of universal life force or *chi,* as we look into our experience with Reiki, a more familiar term is equally accurate: unconditional love. People often arrive at this conclusion after experiencing Reiki: Reiki is love and love is the healer.

Because Reiki's ease of implementation allows delivery of universal life force to wherever it is needed to enhance the overall balance of the individual, Reiki offers many options for physical healing as well as personal growth. With this method of using universal life force to nurture ourselves on all levels, we give ourselves the choice of ever greater mental acuity, emotional stability, and physical heartiness. The use of Reiki supports us in making choices that empower us to develop, evolve, and express ourselves fully, becoming increasingly whole as we do the work we were born to do.

In spite of our technological and scientific advances, we have yet to harness our full potential as human beings. Reiki is a powerful vehicle for conducting an inquiry into the vast knowledge of our inner and outer worlds. The more we do Reiki, the more it benefits us. The actual practice of Reiki caring touch allows our collective consciousness to remember this basic instinct, the remembrance of which is a vital evolutionary piece of our human community. When we marry our sensate awareness with our intellectual knowing, we come into deeper resonance with ourselves and others. Through our physical body we can know the reality of the concepts of quantum physics. Every cell in our body is in vibratory pulsation; every cell in both the animate and inanimate universe is also vibrating. As we become aware of this vibration within ourselves, we become aware of our interrelatedness to all that is. The resulting sense of connection and harmony creates an alignment which is essential among human beings who coinhabit the planet. Reiki enables us to live life with a deeper understanding of what it means to be human: to increase our self-knowledge and self-acceptance, to act with compassion toward ourself and others, and to immerse ourselves in uplifting thoughts and actions. Consistent use of Reiki to increase our self-awareness can lead to the ultimate recognition and experience that we are universal life force.

This experience of our authentic power sets the stage for a

new way to relate to the world. Our sense of wholeness means we no longer need to look to others to fill us. We have a new-found freedom to accept others as they are without the desire to control or manipulate. Out of our state of fullness, we naturally desire to contribute our creative energies and ideas toward making a difference for ourselves and others. Using Reiki consciously with the intention that transformation happens puts less emphasis on doing and more emphasis on allowing and being. There is tremendous power in being aware in the moment. Because we are a microcosm of our universe, as we use Reiki to nurture ourselves, we consciously participate in bringing balance and harmony into our environment as well. In this way Reiki gives each one of us the power to support evolution on a planetary level. Using Reiki as a tool to open the depths of our creative life-giving potential is imperative for transforming the way life is lived on the planet.

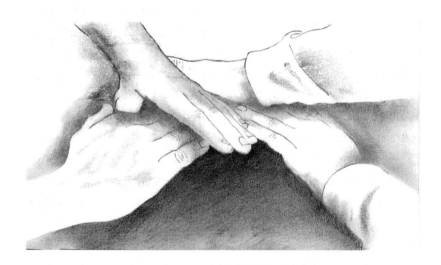

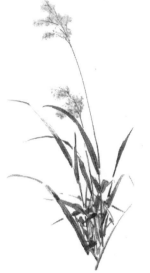

SELF-REIKI
TREATMENT SERIES

The hand positions illustrated in this appendix constitute a traditional Reiki self-treatment practice. While this practice as shown provides you with a form to follow, any and all positions are optional. In order for these Reiki positions to be effective, you must have received the Reiki initiations.

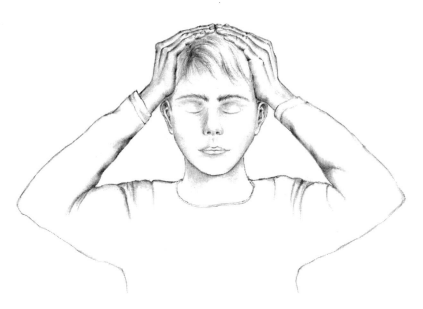

1. Hands rest on top of the head, fingertips touching.

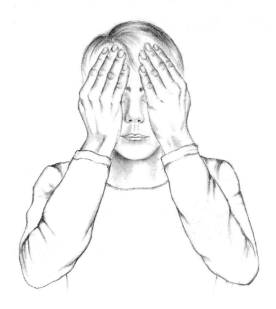

2. Together and slightly cupped, hands rest gently over the eyes, fingers resting on the forehead near the hairline, palms covering the eyes.

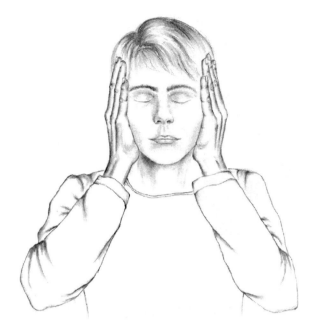

3. Hands are placed on the sides of the head, fingers
   covering the temples, palms holding the lower jaw,
   thumbs behind the ears. Variation: cover the ears.

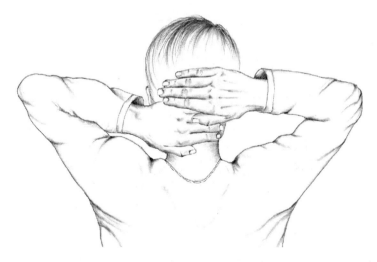

4. Hands cradle the back of the head at the base of the
   skull, being placed horizontally behind the head. One
   hand is above the occipital ridge and rests on the
   other hand below the ridge.

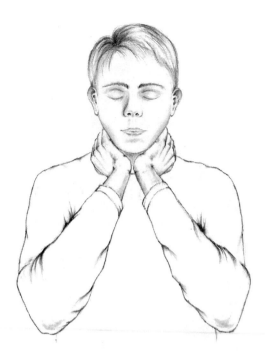

5. Hands cover the throat, heels touching, fingers wrapping around the neck.

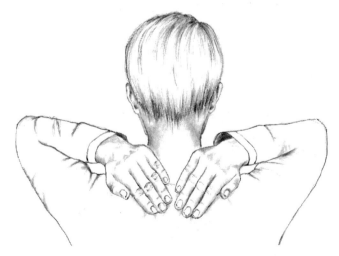

6. Hands cover the top of the shoulders close to the neck.

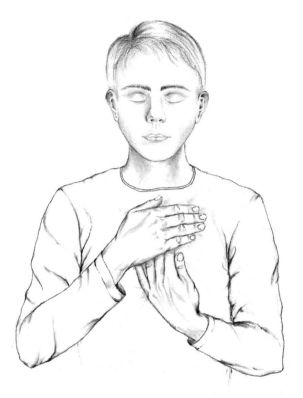

7. Hands form a T, left hand covering the heart, right
   hand covering the thymus.

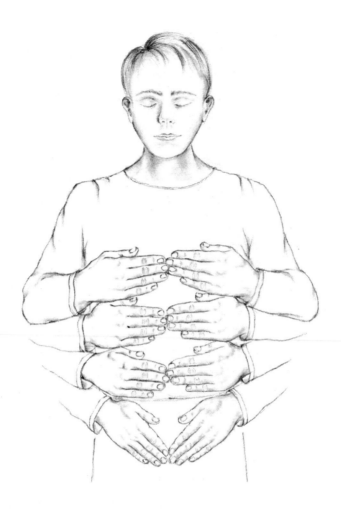

8–11. Hands are placed horizontally in front at the top of the torso, fingertips touching. Hands repeat this position, moving down as many times as necessary to cover the torso, ending in a V inside the hip bones.

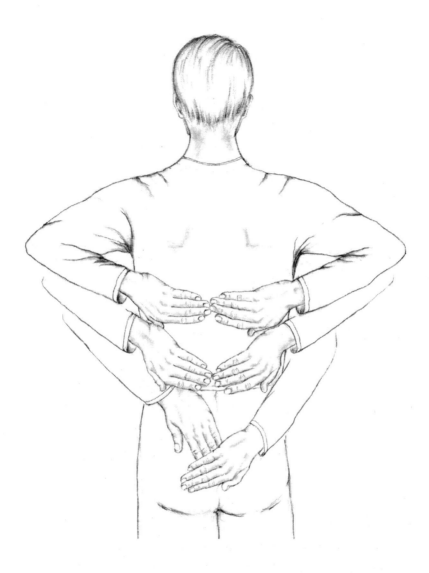

12–15. Hands are horizontal at the back above the waist, fingertips touching. Hands repeat this position, moving down as many times as necessary to cover the back, ending with an upside-down T over the base of the spine.

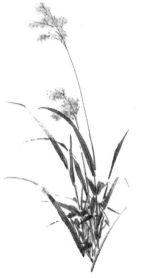

Appendix II

REIKI TREATMENT
ON OTHERS

The hand positions illustrated in this appendix constitute a traditional Reiki treatment for use on others. While this practice as shown provides you with a form to follow, any and all positions are optional. In order for these Reiki positions to be effective, you must have received the Reiki initiations.

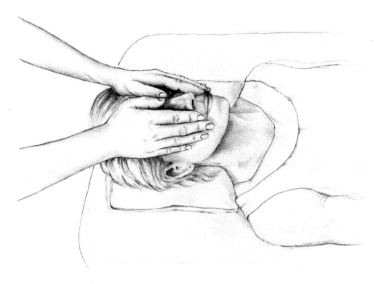

Head

1. With thumbs together, hands rest gently over the eyes, heels resting on forehead, fingers resting on cheekbones.

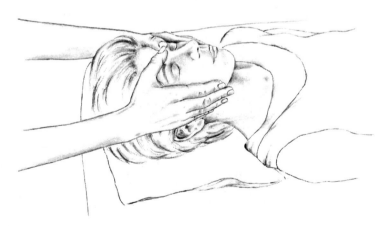

2. Hands are placed on the side of the head, palms covering the temples, fingers covering the jaw. Variation: cover the ears.

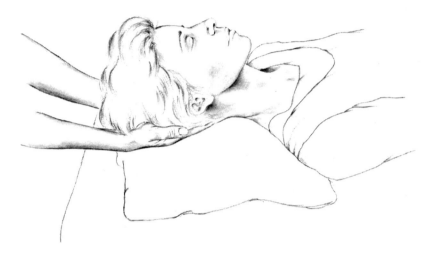

3. Held close together, hands cradle the back of the head, fingertips at the occiput.

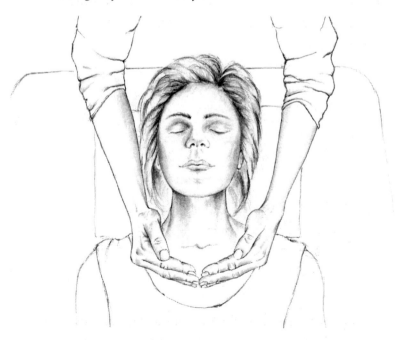

4. Outside edge of hands rest on the collarbone at a 45° angle to the throat.

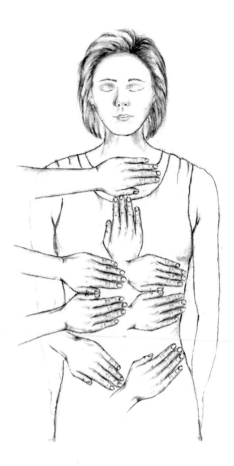

Front

5. Held close together, the hands rest on the left side of the solar plexus below the breastbone.

6. Hands rest as above on the right side of the solar plexus.

7. Hands on the lower abdomen, fingertips of the right hand inside the client's left hip, heel of the left hand inside the client's right hip. Fingertips of the left hand touch heel of the right hand.

8. Left hand horizontal at top of client's chest, covering thymus. Right hand perpendicular to left hand, covering the heart, with fingertips touching left hand.

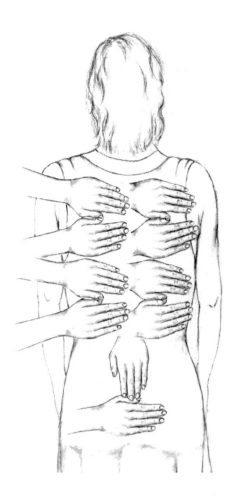

Back

9. Hands cover the top right shoulder blade.
10. Hands cover the top left shoulder blade.
11. Hands cover the mid-back on the right side.
12. Hands cover the mid-back on the left side.
13. Finish with hands in an upside-down T over the coccyx.

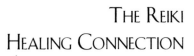

THE REIKI
HEALING CONNECTION

𝒴our body has the capacity to heal itself. However, the ability to consistently tap into the source of this healing has been largely unknown in our society. Reiki is a way for you to connect with your healing ability, restoring balance and harmony to the physical, mental, and emotional levels of your being. Out of our experience that Reiki is essential to optimal well-being, we are dedicated to making Reiki available to all who seek wholeness, love, and connection. For information about our Reiki classes or to schedule a class in your area please contact us.

Libby Barnett, MSW, and Maggie Chambers
Reiki Masters
The Reiki Healing Connection
633 Isaac Frye Highway
Wilton, NH 03086
Phone: (603) 654-2787
Fax: (603) 654-2771
Email: reiki@reikienergy.com
Web page: http://www.reikienergy.com

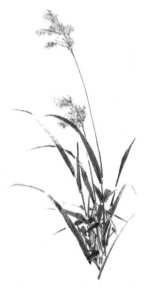

NOTES

FOREWORD

1. Peabody, F. W. *Journal of the American Medical Association* 88 (1927): 877–82.
2. Remen, R. "Working in the Gray Zone: The Dilemma of the Private Practitioner." *Advances* 7 (1991): 3.
3. Dossey, L. "Whatever Happened to Healers?" *Alternative Therapies* 1 (1995): 5.

CHAPTER 1

1. Chopra, Deepak. *Ageless Body, Timeless Mind.* New York: Crown, 1993, 5.
2. Eisenberg, David, et al. "Unconventional Medicine in the United States." *New England Journal of Medicine* 328, no. 4 (1993): 246–52.

CHAPTER 2

1. Wetzel, Wendy S. "Reiki Healing: A Physiologic Perspective and Implications for Nursing." Thesis submitted to Sonoma State University, 1988.
2. Gerber, Richard. *Vibrational Medicine.* Santa Fe, N.M.: Bear and Company, 1988, 371.
3. Brennan, Barbara Ann. *Hands of Light.* New York: Bantam, 1987, 40.

CHAPTER 5

1. Eisenberg, David, et al. "Unconventional Medicine in the United States." *New England Journal of Medicine* 328, no. 4 (1993), 246–52.
2. National Institutes of Health, Technology Assessment Conferences Statement, Integration of Behavioral and Relaxation Approaches into the Treatment of Chronic Pain and Insomnia, October 16–18, 1995.
3. University of Arizona School of Medicine, Center for Integrative Medicine, correspondence, October 1995.
4. Ibid.
5. Brown, Chip. "The Experiments of Dr. Oz." *New York Times Magazine* (July 30, 1995): 21–23.
6. Ibid.
7. Wellspring Cancer Help Program brochure.
8. McCue, Jack. "The Naturalness of Dying." *JAMA* 273, no. 13 (1995): 1039–1043.

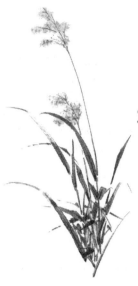

SUGGESTED READING

Baginski, B. J., and Sharamon, S. *Reiki: Universal Life Energy.* Mendocino, Calif.: LifeRhythm, 1988.

Borysenko, Joan, Ph.D. *Minding the Body, Mending the Mind.* Reading, Mass.: Addison-Wesley, 1987.

Brennan, B. A. *Hands of Light.* New York: Bantam Books, 1987.

————. *Light Emerging: The Journey of Personal Healing.* New York: Bantam Books, 1993.

Brown, Fran. *Living Reiki: Takata's Teachings.* Mendocino, Calif.: LifeRhythm, 1992.

Capra, F. *The Tao of Physics,* 2nd ed. New York: Bantam Books, 1984.

Chopra, Deepak, M.D. *Ageless Body, Timeless Mind.* New York: Crown, 1993.

Dossey, Larry, M.D. *Space, Time and Medicine.* Boston: Shambhala Publications, 1985.

————. *Healing Words: The Power of Prayer and the Practice of Medicine.* San Francisco: HarperSanFrancisco, 1993.

Eos, Nancy. *Reiki and Medicine.* Grass Lake, Mich.: Nancy Eos, M.D, 1995.

Gerber, R. *Vibrational Medicine: New Choices for Healing Ourselves.* Santa Fe, N.M.: Bear and Company, 1988.

Haberly, Helen J. *Hawayo Takata's Story.* Olney, Md.: Archedigm Publications, 1990.

Horan, Paula. *Empowerment Through Reiki,* 2nd ed. Wilmot, Wis.: Lotus Light, 1992.

Joy, W. Brugh, M.D. *Joy's Way*. Los Angeles: J. P. Tarcher, 1979.

Kabat-Zinn, Jon, Ph.D. *Full Catastrophe Living*. New York: Delta, 1991.

Levine, Stephen. *Healing into Life and Death*. New York: Anchor Books, 1987.

Moyers, Bill. *Healing and the Mind*. New York: Doubleday, 1993.

Myss, Carolyn and Shealy, Norm. *Creation of Health*. Walpole, N.H.: Stillpoint Publishing, 1993

Rinpoche, Sogyal. *The Tibetan Book of Living and Dying*. San Francisco: HarperSanFrancisco, 1992.

Seigel, Bernie S., M.D. *Love, Medicine and Miracles*. New York: Harper and Row, 1986.

Stewart, Judy-Carol. *Reiki Touch*. Houston, Tex.: The Reiki Touch, Inc., 1995.

Zukav, Gary. *The Dancing Wu Li Masters*. New York: Bantam Books, 1979.

———. *The Seat of the Soul*. New York: Simon and Schuster, 1989.

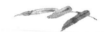

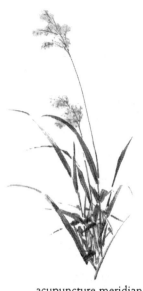

INDEX

Lister, Joseph, 11–12
Massachusetts General Hospital, 6–7, 30, 79, 88
    Mind-Body Medicine Group at, 7, 90
massage, 51, 93
McCue, Jack, 100
Medical Center of Central Massachusetts (The), 2, 11
Medical Revolution (The), 7–12
meditation, 26, 93
Mind/Body Medical Institute, 91
Moyers, Bill, 8. *See also* "Healing and the Mind," (PBS television series)
Mutual of Omaha, 94
National Institutes of Health, 9. *See also* Office of Alternative Medicine (The);
    Office of Medical Applications of Research (The)
nature, 26
New England Journal of Medicine (The), 9
New London Hospital, 2
Northrup, Christiane, 8
Office of Alternative Medicine (The), 9, 16, 89, 91
Office of Medical Applications of Research (The), 89
Ornish, Dean, 94
Oz, Mehmet, 8, 92
Pardes, Herbert, 92
particles (subatomic), 19
pelvic exams, 62
Pettinati, Pamela, 19, 63–64
pharmacologic intervention, 57
physicists, 13–14
physics, 19–20, 23, 44
prana, 1–2
psychotherapy, 54, 76–84
Reiki, 1–34
    anecdotes concerning:
        ankle injury, 23–25
        brain tumor, 59–60, 61
        bone marrow transplant, 57
        child-abuse survivors, 77–79
        detached retina, 58
        dying, 72–74
    emotional patterns, 31
    fibroid tumor, 52
    head trauma, 17–18, 31
    hernia, 4–5
    hysterectomy, 61–62
        incest survivor(s), 81
    intimacy, 82
    intuition and creativity, 30
    anecdotes concerning:
        low self-esteem, 76–77
        neurological damage, 70–71
        pain, 71–72

Reiki (continued),
  anecdotes concerning (continued):
    vertebrae (crushed), 29
  and the caregiving team, 95–97
  clinics, 97
  and community outreach, 97–98
  four initiations of, 27–33
  misdiagnosis with, 22
  practitioners of, 22, 32, 40
  resolution technique (the), 43–49
  self-treatment protocol, 37–43, 105–111
  students of, 15, 22, 27–28, 66, 81
  treatment on others, 113–117
Richard and Hinda Rosenthal Center for Alternative/Complementary
  Medicine, 92
Rothfeld, Glenn, 91
Rufsvold, Bob, 91, 94
Saint Elizabeth's Medical Center (Boston), 19
Sanskrit texts, 27
Savage, Seddon, 91
Self-Reiki, 35–49, 98
  resolving emotional patterns with, 43–49
  treatment series, 105–111
Siegel, Bernie, 8
Simmons College School of Social Work, 79
sleep, 39
Sonoma State University, 16
Southern New Hampshire Medical Center, 2
tai chi, 92
Takata, Hawayo, 14, 27
therapeutic touch, 51
Tufts University School of Medicine. See Humanistic and Holistic Health Care
  (organization)
universal life force (the), 14, 16, 20, 23, 32, 40, 46, 48, 52, 58, 62–63, 70, 101.
  See also chi; life-force energy
University of Arizona School of Medicine. See Center for Integrative Medicine
  (The)
University of Virginia School of Medicine (The), 90
Usui, Mikao, 2, 6, 14, 27
Vibrational Medicine, 21
visualization, 51
VNA of the Greater Milford/Northbridge Area, 2
Weil, Andrew, 8, 90–91
Wellspring Cancer Help Program, 93
Wellspring Foundation of New England, 94
Wentworth-Douglass Hospital, 3
Wetzel, Wendy, 16
yoga, 93